SpringerBriefs in Cancer Res

More information about this series at http://www.springer.com/series/10786

Michael J. Gonzalez · Jorge R. Miranda-Massari

New Insights on Vitamin C and Cancer

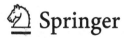 Springer

Michael J. Gonzalez
Department of Human Development
Nutrition Program
School of Public Health
Medical Sciences Campus
University of Puerto Rico
San Juan
Puerto Rico

Jorge R. Miranda-Massari
Department Pharmacy Practice
School of Pharmacy
Medical Sciences Campus
University of Puerto Rico
San Juan
Puerto Rico

ISBN 978-1-4939-1889-8   ISBN 978-1-4939-1890-4   (eBook)
DOI 10.1007/978-1-4939-1890-4

Library of Congress Control Number: 2014949331

Springer New York Heidelberg Dordrecht London

Printed on acid-free paper

Springer is part of Springer Science+Business Media (www.springer.com)

Preface

It is a privilege bestowed upon us to write this book on Vitamin C and Cancer. It is humbling for us to follow in the steps of scientific giants such as Nobel Prize winner Hungarian physiologist, Dr. Albert Szent-Görgyi, American Medical Researcher Dr. Frederick R. Klenner, the great American scientist Dr. Linus C. Pauling, two time (Unshared) Nobel Prize winner, distinguished Scottish surgeon, Dr. Ewan Cameron, prominent Canadian psychiatrist, Dr. Abram Hoffer, outstanding American ortho-molecular physician, Dr. Hugh D. Riordan, and leading NIH medical scientist, Dr. Mark Levine; all brave medical mavericks that have been key to the development of the science behind Vitamin C and Cancer. It is a great honor to follow in the steps of these inquisitive and bright scientists. Nowadays, Dr. Neil H. Riordan, Dr. Steve Hickey, Dr. Ron Hunninghake, Dr. Atsuo Yanagisawa, Dr. Chan H. Park, Dr. Qi Chen, Dr. Sebastian J. Padayatti, Dr. Chang H. Yeom, Dr. Thomas Levy, Dr. Nina Mikirova, Dr. Joseph Casciari, Dr. Jorge Duconge, and Dr. Jeanne Drisko continue to study and research Vitamin C and Cancer to provide valuable information regarding its therapeutic use as Cancer therapy.

We embark on this project with humility but with a special personal interest since we both have suffered personal losses due to Cancer. Dr. Miranda's wife, mother, and father and Dr. Gonzalez's mother, grandmother, and grandfather, all have succumbed to the devastation of Cancer. In this sense any opportunity we have to study, understand, and fight Cancer, we will seize. Moreover, any chance to contribute to improve survival and quality of life of Cancer patients, is not only welcomed but sought after.

Vitamin C and Cancer has been a subject of much controversy. We think the main reason for this dispute has been a lack of knowledge probably due to lack of reliable scientific information. We should add to this that most available informa-tion on the subject are case reports and clinical observations or experiences lacking proper scientific follow-up. We hope to contribute with this book in trying to fulfill such need and at the same time provide some light on the existing debate on its use as an adjuvant in Cancer therapy.

Well without further preamble…

Here we go…

Michael J. Gonzalez
Jorge R. Miranda-Massari

Contents

Chapter 1
Overview of Vitamin C and Cancer

History of Vitamin C: A Briefing

In 1536, the French explorer Jacques Cartier, while exploring the St. Lawrence River, used the local natives' herbal medicine knowledge to save his men who were dying of scurvy. He boiled the needles of the arbor vitae tree to make the healing tea (that was later shown to contain about 50 mg of vitamin C per 100 g) [1].

In the winter of the year 1556, there was a scurvy epidemic that plagued Europe. A lack of fruits and vegetables in those cold winter months had caused the outbreak. While this was one of the earliest documented scurvy epidemics, not much research was done in effort to understand, more less cure this disease until many centuries later.

The earliest documented case of scurvy was described by Hippocrates around the year 400 BC, but the first attempt to provide a scientific basis for the cause of this disease was by British Royal Navy ship's surgeon, Dr. James Lind. Scurvy was common among those with poor access to fresh fruit and vegetables, such as remote, isolated sailors, and soldiers. While at sea in May 1747, Dr. Lind provided some crew members with two oranges and one lemon per day, in addition to normal rations, while others continued on cider, vinegar, sulfuric acid, or seawater, along with their normal rations. In the history of science, this is considered to be the first controlled experiment comparing results on two populations with a factor applied to one group only with all other factors remaining the same. The results conclusively demonstrated that citrus fruits prevented the disease. Dr. Lind published his work in 1753 in his "Treatise on the Scurvy" [2].

In 1912, the Polish American biochemist Dr. Casimir Funk, while researching deficiency diseases, developed the concept of vitamins to refer to the non-mineral micronutrients which are essential for health. The name is a combination of "vital," due to the vital role they play biochemically, and "amines" because Dr. Funk thought that all these chemicals were amines. One of the "vitamins" was thought to be the antiscorbutic factor, long thought to be a component of fresh plant material.

© The Author(s) 2014   1
M.J. Gonzalez and J.R. Miranda-Massari, *New Insights on Vitamin C and Cancer*,
SpringerBriefs in Cancer Research, DOI 10.1007/978-1-4939-1890-4_1

From 1928 to 1933, the Hungarian research team of Dr. Joseph L Svirbely and Dr. Albert Szent-Györgyi and, independently, the American scientist Dr. Charles Glen King first isolated the antiscorbutic factor, calling it "ascorbic acid." Ascorbic acid was not an amine, nor even contained any nitrogen. Dr. Szent-Györgyi was awarded the 1937 Nobel Prize in Medicine "for his discoveries in connection with the biological combustion processes, with special reference to vitamin C and the catalysis of fumaric acid" [3].

Between 1933 and 1934, the British chemists Sir Walter Norman Haworth and Sir Edmund Hirst and, independently, the Polish chemist Dr. Tadeus Reichstein succeeded in synthesizing the vitamin, making it the first vitamin to be artificially produced. This made possible the cheap mass production of vitamin C. Haworth was awarded the 1937 Nobel Prize in Chemistry for this work.

In 1933, Hoffmann La Roche became the first pharmaceutical company to mass-produce synthetic vitamin C, under the brand name of Redoxon.

In 1957, the American scientist Dr. J. J. Burns showed that the reason some mammals were susceptible to scurvy was the inability of their liver to produce the active enzyme L-gulonolactone oxidase, which is the last in the chain of four enzymes which synthesize vitamin C. American biochemist Dr. Irwin Stone was the first to use vitamin C for its food preservative properties. He later developed the theory that humans possess a mutated form of the L-gulonolactone oxidase coding gene. Dr. Stone wrote in 1972, the book "The Healing Factor: Vitamin C Against Disease" [4]. In 1952 Vitamin C was first proposed as a chemotherapeutic agent by McCormick [5].

General Mechanisms of Vitamin C

Biochemistry of Vitamin C

Vitamin C (ascorbic acid, ascorbate C_6, H_{12}, O_6) is a six-carbon ketolactone with a molecular weight of 176.13 g/ml which is synthesized from glucose by many animals. Vitamin C is synthesized in the liver in some mammals and in the kidney in birds and reptiles. However, several species, including humans, non-human primates, guinea pigs, and Indian fruit bats, are unable to synthesize vitamin C. When there is insufficient vitamin C in the diet, humans suffer from the potentially lethal deficiency disease scurvy. Humans and primates lack the terminal enzyme in the biosynthetic pathway of ascorbic acid, l-gulonolactone oxidase. Vitamin C is an electron donor (reducing agent or antioxidant). Vitamin C acts as an electron donor for eight enzymes.

A basic biochemical role for ascorbic acid (ascorbate, AA) is to accelerate hydroxylation reactions in a number of biosynthetic pathways. In many of these reactions, ascorbate directly or indirectly provides electrons to enzymes that require prosthetic metal ions in a reduced form to achieve full enzymatic activity. The best known biochemical role of ascorbate is that of cofactor for prolyl and lysyl

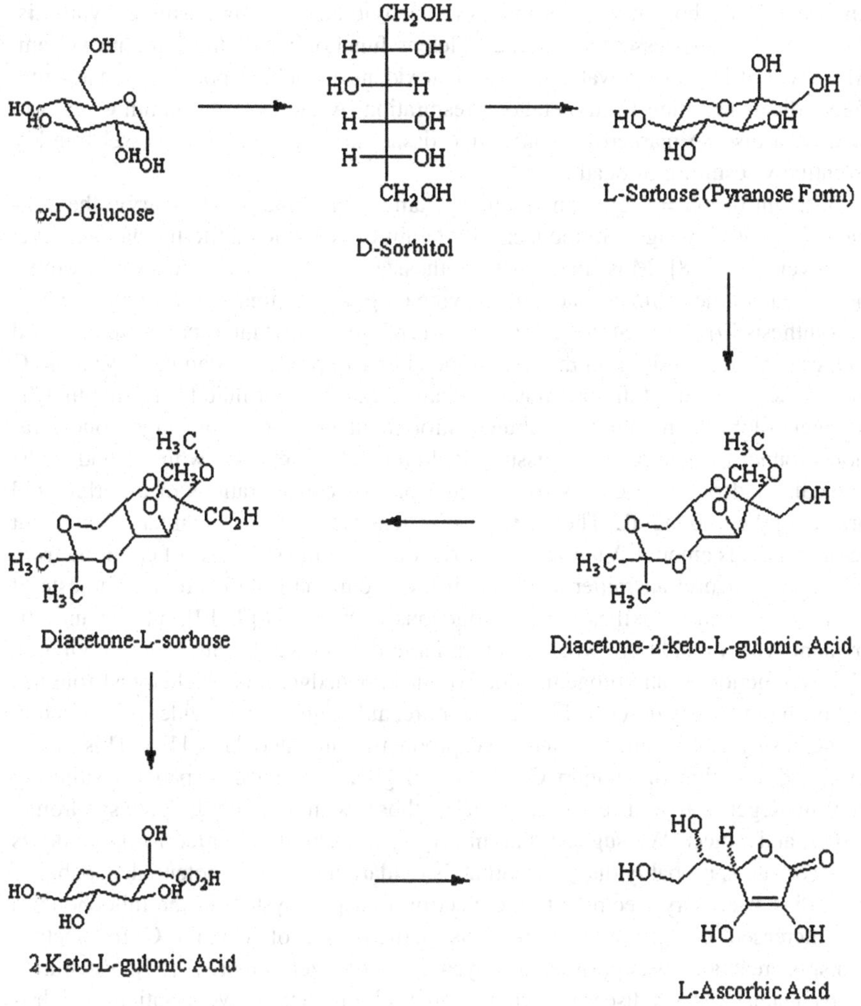

Fig. 1.1 Glucose conversion to ascorbic acid sequence

hydroylase enzymes in the biosynthesis of collagen [6]. The molecular structures of ascorbic acid and its oxidized form dihydroascorbic acid are similar to that of glucose (see Fig. 1.1).

Biological Functions of Vitamin C

Vitamin C was isolated by Szent-Györgyi in 1928. The vitamin plays a key role in several biological functions including the biosynthesis of collagen and L-carnitine, cholesterol metabolism, cytochrome P-450 activity, and neurotransmitter synthesis. Vitamin C is also essential for the efficient functioning of the immune system. Moreover, it is a major water-soluble antioxidant quenching potentially damaging free radicals resulting from metabolic respiration. Acute lack of vitamin C leads to scurvy, a disease marked by connective tissue damage and blood vessel fragility eventually resulting in death.

Vitamin C (pk = 4.2) is an essential vitamin for humans [7]. Scurvy, the deficiency disease arising from the lack of vitamin C, can reach a life-threatening level and even death [8]. Most mammals synthesize ascorbate from glucose; however, humans and other primates lack the enzyme (L-gulonolactone oxidase) required for its synthesis [9]. Irwin Stone proposed, in 1965, that a mutation may have occurred in these species resulting in the loss of the ability to produce vitamin C. Vitamin C is considered the most important antioxidant in extracellular fluid [10]. Vitamin C is a water-soluble compound distributed throughout the body, with high concentrations found in a number of tissues including the eye lens, white blood cells, adrenals, and pituitary glands [6]. Normal plasma concentrations of ascorbic acid are about 0.6–2.0 mg/dL. These tissues (eye lens, adrenals, and pituitary) contain at least twice this amount. Vitamin C is also required in the synthesis of carnitine from lysine [11], neurotransmitter synthesis [6], cytochrome P-450 activity, cholesterol metabolism, and detoxification of exogenous compounds [9, 12], and as an antioxidant [10]. In addition, when given in large doses (mainly intravenous), vitamin C may function as an ergogenic aid. To our knowledge, this biochemical role has not been previously described in the literature, although there is evidence of vitamin C increasing cell respiration and ATP production in osteoblasts [13]. This newly proposed function of vitamin C may be of great relevance to patients suffering chronic-degenerative diseases, especially those with chronic fatigue syndrome, AIDS, and cancer. We suggest that this ergogenic activity reported for large doses of ascorbate is probably due to ascorbate's oxidation reduction potential, capable of providing necessary electrons to the electron transport system in the mitochondria for increased energy production. This participation of vitamin C in electron transport reactions was postulated 71 years ago by Szent-Gyorgyi [14]. Vitamin C helps against various diseases such as diabetes by reducing glycolysation, which is an abnormal attachment of sugars to proteins [15].

Aspects of Vitamin C Dosing

Dosing Vitamin C: The Evolutionary Perspective

Ever since Albert Szent-Györgyi first isolated ascorbic acid and identified it as vitamin C in the late 1920s, controversy has ensued. There is continuing debate within the scientific community over the best dose schedule (the amount and frequency of intake) of vitamin C for maintaining optimal health in humans.

People seem to vary widely in their requirements for vitamin C. The RDA for vitamin C is based on twice the amount of vitamin C needed to prevent scurvy as well as on the threshold of the vitamin C needed to spill vitamin C into urinary excretion. Moreover, the RDA for vitamin C is based on estimates of vitamin C absorption, on losses associated with food preparation, and on estimated rates of depletion, turnover, and catabolism. Levine postulated that to establish an RDA for a vitamin, it is necessary to determine vitamin concentrations in plasma and tissues. Initially, the RDA for vitamin C was based on the amount needed to prevent people from getting scurvy with a safety margin but this may not lead to optimal health.

The current RDA of 60 mg/d is clearly far too low, and the proposed new RDA of 200 mg/d while perhaps may be adequate for healthy, young males would seem to be quite inadequate for older people and certainly too low for sick people.

Irwin Stone, Linus Pauling, and others have argued that the level of vitamin C intake needed to promote optimal health is far greater than the RDA and far greater than the amount found in a typical diet. To support this argument, Stone pointed out that humans are among a small group of species that are unable to synthesize vitamin C. Stone named this genetic defect hypoascorbemia, in reference to the abnormally low levels of vitamin C that can exist in species that are unable to synthesize vitamin C. He hypothesized that "full correction" of this inborn error of metabolism would require supplying the individual with as much vitamin C as the liver would be synthesizing if the genetic defect was not present. It is possible that some benefit can be derived from having the blood and tissues saturated with vitamin C and from large amounts of the vitamin being excreted in the urine and sweat. For example, because vitamin C has anti-viral and anti-bacterial activity, excretion of large amounts in the urine and sweat might help prevent urinary tract and cutaneous infections.

Researchers skeptical of the value of high-dose vitamin C have pointed out that when vitamin C intake is high, further increases in intake produce only small increases in plasma or tissue levels of the vitamin. However, as suggested by Pauling, the human body might be sensitive to small changes in plasma or tissue vitamin C levels. There are many examples of substances in body fluids for which a 10–25 % change in concentration has clinical consequences, e.g., glucose, sodium, calcium, chloride, and hemoglobin. Therefore, the absence of dramatic changes in plasma and tissue vitamin C levels does not rule out the possibility that large doses of the vitamin can be beneficial.

Vitamin C intake has been found to speed resolution of upper respiratory tract infections in young people. Students who supplemented with hourly doses of 1,000 mg of vitamin C for 6 h and then three times daily thereafter exhibited an extraordinary 85 % decrease in cold and flu symptoms compared to those who took pain relievers and decongestants for their infectious symptoms [16]. These benefits of improved healing are not limited to children and young adults. Elderly patients that were hospitalized with pneumonia or bronchitis showed substantial improvement following supplementation with vitamin C [17]. Dr. Steve Hickey proposed in 2005 an elegant model of Vitamin C pharmacokinetics, the dynamic Flow in which a specific oral dosing scheme achieve the maximal blood concentrations [18].

Rethinking the Classical Vitamin C and Cancer Controversy

In the late 1970s and early 1980s, a debate ensued between Dr. Linus Pauling (Linus Pauling Institute) and Dr. Charles Moertel (Mayo Clinic) due to conflicting results on studies on vitamin C and cancer [19–21]. To make the story short, the Pauling and Cameron studies utilized historical controls and were positive, while the Mayo Clinic studies were done in a prospective randomized double-blinded fashion and had negative results. The Mayo Clinic studies were done with the accepted experimental design used to clarify initial observations, but did not truly replicate the Cameron and Pauling studies (used a lesser dosage, less time). This issue has been reviewed elsewhere [22].

A critical point of both studies (Mayo Clinic and Pauling's) is that they used oral doses of ascorbate of about 10 g. Given the saturable gastrointestinal absorption and the nonlinear renal clearance [23], oral absorption of vitamin C cannot achieve plasma concentrations comparable to those obtained by intravenous administration [24]. Plasma concentrations of ascorbic acid rise as the dose ingested increases until a plateau is reached with doses of about 150–200 mg daily.

Moreover, there is a recent report on vitamin C as a toxic agent against cancer cells when given intravenously [25]. The doses we are advocating for therapy are substantially higher doses (25–200 g) and most importantly are given intravenously. We believe intravenous administration is more effective, because plasma levels of ascorbate can reach higher levels than those attained by oral intakes and these higher levels can be sustained for longer periods of time. These two aspects seem necessary to produce a selective toxic effect by vitamin C on cancer cells. We are attempting to reach plasma levels that are 100 times higher than those that can be achieved by oral administration.

Contradictory Data on Vitamin C and Cancer

There are some seemingly contradictory studies regarding the effect of vitamin C (Ascobic Acid, AA) and its effect on cancer cells. AA has been reported to enhance chemical carcinogenesis in a rodent model [26–28]. This action may be due to the pro-oxidant activity of AA and the subsequent enhancement of free radical formation by the chemical carcinogen 7,12-dimethylbenz[a]anthracene (DMBA). In another study, AA in low concentrations was found to be an essential requirement for the growth of murine myeloma cells in cell culture [29]. In contrast, further studies by the same group reported that AA inhibited growth at higher concentrations [30]. Also, Vitamin C at low doses (± 25 µg/mL) without any other added antioxidants has been reported to stimulate growth of malignant cells, while inhibiting their growth at higher doses (± 200 µg/mL) [31]. These studies constitute a very important contribution in terms of understanding AA dose effect on malignant cells. In addition, these studies help determine a therapeutic dosing range of AA for cancer, specifically the proper dose and the concomitant use of synergistic nutrients. Therefore, instead of being contradictory, these studies actually reinforce the importance of using high-dose AA to achieve a chemotherapeutic effect.

Intravenous Vitamin C Essentials

General Information on Intravenous Vitamin C

Physiological concentrations of vitamin C (L-ascorbate or L-ascorbic acid) in the body are controlled through intestinal absorption, tissue accumulation, and renal reabsorption and excretion. Therefore, intravenous administration is used to achieve pharmacologic doses not attainable by other means.

In relation to cancer, high-dose intravenous vitamin C (>0.5 g/kg body weight) has several effects: (a) cytotoxicity for cancer cells, but not for normal cells, (b) improved quality of life for cancer patients, (c) protection of normal tissues from toxicity caused by chemotherapy, (d) reinforcement of the action of radiation and some types of chemotherapy, (e) immune system enhancement, and (f) strengthening of collagen and hyaluronic acid.

To date, no randomized controlled clinical trial with high-dose intravenous vitamin C as cancer therapy has been published. A number of Phase I clinical trials (see section on Phase 1 studies) confirm the non-toxic nature of the treatment and give indications of improvement in quality of life (see section on quality of life). Several case reports show a positive effect on survival time, even showing cancer remission (see section on case reports).

High-dose vitamin C is essentially non-toxic. Reported side effects are minor if patients are adequately screened for renal disease and glucose 6-phosphate dehydrogenase deficiency and when doses are gradually increased with careful monitoring of the patient.

Application and Dosage

Vitamin C can be administered via several routes including orally. This treatise only discusses the intravenous administration of high doses of vitamin C (>0.5 g/kg body weight).

Phase 1 dose-finding studies recommend the use of 1.5 g intravenous vitamin C per kg body weight three times weekly. In further clinical research, it is advised to start treatment with a lower dose, and, if no adverse events are observed, to gradually increase doses to their final desired level [32–34]. The dose of 1.5 g/kg body weight was found to be safe and to be capable of achieving plasma ascorbic acid concentrations of more than 10 mM for several hours in patients with normal renal function.

Ascorbic acid solutions for clinical infusion might be unstable over time, especially if given in conjunction with B complex [35–37].

In the late 1990s, it was found that vitamin C concentrations in plasma and tissues were tightly controlled through intestinal absorption, tissue accumulation, and renal reabsorption and excretion [38–40]. As a result, it was very difficult to increase plasma and tissue concentrations with oral intakes of vitamin C. However, intravenous administration bypassed this tight control until equilibrium was restored through renal excretion. In healthy volunteers, oral administration of the maximum tolerated dose of 3 g every 4 h resulted in peak plasma concentrations of 0.22 mM, while an intravenous vitamin C dose of 50 g produced a peak plasma concentration of 13.4 mM [41]. Comparable results were found in cancer patients [32, 42, 43].

Hence, the IV route of administration is critical in achieving pharmacologic concentrations of vitamin C needed to attain antineoplastic activity, which calls for a re-evaluation of vitamin C in cancer treatment [44].

Most Relevant Mechanism(s) of Action

At low physiological concentrations (0.1 mM), vitamin C works as antioxidant that inactivates reactive oxygen species [45]. However, at high pharmacologic concentrations (up to 20 mM), it was found to have a pro-oxidant action generating oxidative species, i.e., extracellular hydrogen peroxide, which is lethal to cancer cells [46, 47]. Normal cells were unaffected by both concentrations of vitamin C. In vitro findings were confirmed in rats and mice, where virtually the same cancer-killing hydrogen peroxide concentrations were found in extracellular fluid, but not in blood, after intravenous administration of high-dose vitamin C, oral doses did not result in generation of hydrogen peroxide [48–50]. It was proposed that extracellular hydrogen peroxide diffuses into cancer cells and mediates toxicity by ATP depletion, thereby causing cell death. Moreover, hydrogen peroxide toxicity compromises membranes, glucose metabolism, and DNA integrity. In normal cells, hydrogen peroxide is readily neutralized by antioxidant enzymes such as catalase, gluthatione peroxidase, and superoxide dismutase, while levels of these antioxidant enzymes are low or imbalanced in most human cancers [51]. (For other mechanisms, see references on Chap. 8).

Daily high-dose intravenous vitamin C significantly decreased the volume of tumors in mice by 41–53 % for diverse aggressive cancer types [49]. Inhibition of tumor growth was also found in other mouse models of human cancers and human cancer cell lines [50, 52–57].

Prevalence of Use

Mainstream oncologists do not use high-dose intravenous Vitamin C therapy for cancer, but the compound is in wide use by complementary and alternative medicine practitioners [58].

Cost and Expenditure

Vitamin C infusions, to be applied by a medical practitioner, are widely available at moderate cost ($ 100.00–$ 300.00 per infusion in a clinic).

Adverse Events/Contraindications

Vitamin C itself is essentially non-toxic. In general, adverse events after high-dose intravenous vitamin C were mild [32, 58, 59], consistent with side effects occurring due to rapid infusion of any high-osmolarity solution, and were preventable by drinking water before and during the infusion [32].

Hemolysis in G6PD Deficiency

Patients with glucose 6-phosphate dehydrogenase deficiency were found to be at risk to experience hemolysis (breakdown of red blood cells) following administration of high doses of vitamin C [60, 61]. Patients should therefore be tested for G6PD deficiency before they are given large doses of vitamin C intravenously. The highest prevalence of G6PD deficiency is found in African Americans, Asians, and individuals of Mediterranean descent. While the hemolytic effect of vitamin C in patients with G6PD deficiency seems dose related, it is not known what dosage of intravenous vitamin C would be safe for these individuals. Numerous practitioners administer 1–5 g of vitamin C intravenously as a component of the Myers' cocktail without first testing for G6PD deficiency without any problem. Among the many thousands of patients who have received this treatment, there have been no reports of severe hemolytic episodes. However, it is possible that minor episodes of hemolysis have gone unrecognized.

A concern is life-threatening bleeding (hemorrhage) and rapid necrosis of tumors that may occur in cancer patients given large doses of intravenous vitamin C [62]. Authors therefore advised a slow gradual increase of intravenous vitamin C while monitoring the patient with a high tumor burden. However, in the 28 years of administering intravenous vitamin C at the Center for the Improvement of Human Functioning, they never had an episode of tumor necrosis. Patients may become very ill because their bodies could not cope with the sudden task of getting rid of such a large mass of dead tissue. This is a concern mainly for patients suffering from end-stage disease with a considerable tumor load, and highly aggressive, rapidly dividing tumors. This might be the main reason not to overload the body's detoxification systems (skin, kidneys, colon, and liver) while on vitamin C therapy.

Kidney Stones and Oxalosis

It has frequently been claimed that ingestion of large doses of vitamin C can increase the risk of calcium oxalate kidney stones, because vitamin C is converted in part to oxalate. Oxalic acid is an end product of metabolic oxidation of vitamin C. Oxalate nephropathy has been reported after administration of intravenous vitamin C in subjects with renal dysfunction [63, 64]. However, in people with normal renal function, only about 2 % of large doses intravenous vitamin C (1.5 g/kg body weight) was found in the urine as oxalic acid 6 h after infusion [65]. However, the hyperoxaluria associated with the use of high-dose vitamin C has been found to be due primarily to a laboratory artifact, resulting from the conversion of vitamin C to oxalate ex vivo, i.e., after it has left the body, while it is in the collection bottle. If there is a small increase in urinary oxalate resulting from ingestion of large doses of vitamin C, that increase might be counterbalanced by other effects of the vitamin. For example, vitamin C binds calcium in the urine, potentially reducing the formation of calcium oxalate crystals; produces a small increase in urinary acidity, thereby increasing calcium oxalate solubility; and possibly decreases urinary stasis by promoting diuresis. Various studies have found either that vitamin C intake is not associated with kidney stone risk or that higher intake is associated with a lower incidence of kidney stones [66–71] and found no evidence of vitamin C increasing the risk of kidney stone formation.

Moreover, practitioners who have routinely used large doses of vitamin C have not observed kidney stones as a side effect. Despite the apparent safety of vitamin C for the general population with respect to kidney stone risk, there are rare cases in which high-dose vitamin C appeared to cause an increase in urinary oxalate levels. Hence, in this population, the risk of oxalate crystallization in the kidney was not increased, in particular since calcium oxalate stones develop over months to years. Therefore, research results conclude that high-dose intravenous vitamin C may be contraindicated in people with renal dysfunction, and a history of kidney stones should be reviewed.

General Safety and Toxicity Considerations of High Doses of Vitamin C

Vitamin C is remarkably non-toxic at high levels (10–100 times the RDA when taken po). Nevertheless, some minor toxic effects have been reported. These side effects include acidosis, oxaluria, renal stones, glycosuria, renal tubular disease, gastrointestinal disturbances, sensitivity reactions, conditioned need, prothrombin and cholesterol disturbances, vitamin B12 destruction, fatigue, and sterility [72]. Of these side effects, gastrointestinal disturbances are perhaps the most consistent and prevalent problem following the ingestion of large quantities of oral ascorbic acid since nausea, abdominal cramps, and diarrhea are frequently mentioned as negative side effects. These effects are lessened or eliminated by taking ascorbic acid as a buffered salt or immediately after meals. The amount of oral vitamin C tolerated by a patient without producing diarrhea increases in proportion to the stress or severity of his ailment [73]. Bowel tolerance doses of ascorbic acid ameliorate the acute symptoms of many diseases. Lesser doses often have little effect on acute symptoms, but assist the body in handling the stress of disease and may reduce the morbidity of the disease [74]. Many of the toxic effects reported for taking large amounts of vitamin C in reality are insignificant, rare, and of minor consequences. Also while on vitamin C therapy, intake of inorganic selenium (Na selenite) should be avoided. A possibility exists that ascorbic acid may reduce selenite and render it unavailable for tissue uptake [75].

In relation to vitamin C given intravenously, no ill effects have been reported with doses as high as 150–200 g over a 24-h period [42, 76–81]. Vitamin C is more efficient when administered intravenously than when given orally because it bypasses the gut and higher circulating levels are achieved for longer periods of time. Vitamin C has a unique advantage relative to other currently utilized remedies for cancer, and it is generally harmless and safe even at sustained high doses for prolonged periods of time. Evidence supports the concept of using high-dose intravenous vitamin C for extended periods, in doses high enough to achieve and maintain plasma levels above those which have been found to be preferentially cytotoxic to tumor cells [33, 77, 78]. Vitamin C is one of the safest substances available to the physician.

References

1. Martini E. Jacques Cartier witnesses a treatment for scurvy. Vesalius. 2002;8(1):2–6.
2. Lind J. A treatise of the scurvy: in three parts, containing an inquiry into the nature, causes and cure of that disease, together with a critical and chronological view of what has been published on the subject. London: A. Millar; 1753.
3. Lectures Nobel. Physiology or medicine 1922–1941. Amsterdam: Elsevier Publishing Company; 1965.
4. Stone I. The healing factor: vitamin C against disease. New York: Grosset & Dunlap; 1974.
5. McCormick WJ. Ascorbic acid as a chemotherapeutic agent. Arch Pediat. 1952;69:151–155.
6. Levine M. New concepts in the biology and biochemistry of ascorbic acid. New Engl J Med. 1986;314:892–902.
7. Food and Nutrition Board, National Research Council. Recommended dietary allowances. 10th ed. Washington, DC: Natl Acad Press; 1989.
8. Guthrie H. Introductory nutrition. 7th ed. Missouri: Mosby College Publishing; 1989. pp. 381–382.

9. Shils M. In: Shils M, Olson J and Shike M, editors. Modern nutrition in health and disease. 8th ed. Lea and Febiger; 1994. pp. 444–445.
10. Sies H, Stahl W, Sundquist A. Antioxidants functions of vitamins. Ann NY Acad Sci. 1992;669:7–20.
11. Leibovitz B, Mueller J. Carnitine. J Optimal Nutr. 1993;2:90–109.
12. Block G. Vitamin C and cancer prevention: the epidemiologic evidence. Am J Clin Nutr. 1991;53:270s–82s.
13. Komarova SV, Ataullakhanov FI, Globus RK. Bioenergetics and mitochondrial transmembrane potential during differentiation of cultured osteoblasts. Am J Physiol Cell Physiol. 2000;279:c1220–9.
14. Szent Gyorgyi A. Introduction to submolecular biology. J Biol Chem, 1960; 90:385.
15. Will JC, Tyers T. Does diabetes mellitus increase the requirement for vitamin C? Nutr Rev. 1996;54:193–202.
16. Gorton HC, Jarvis K. The effectiveness of vitamin C in preventing and relieving the symptoms of virus-induced respiratory infections. J Manipulative Physiol Ther. 1999;22(8):530–3.
17. Hemila H, Douglas RM. Vitamin C and acute respiratory infections. Int J Tuberc Lung Dis. 1999;3(9):756–61.
18. Hickey DS, Roberts HJ, Cathcart RF. Dynamic flow: A new model for ascorbate. JOM 2005;20:237–40.
19. Cameron E, Pauling L. Supplemental ascorbate in the supportive treatment of cancer: prolongation of survival times in terminal human cancer. Proc Natl Acad Sci USA. 1976;73:3685–9.
20. Creagan ET, Moertel CG, O'Fallon JR, Schutt AJ, O'Connell MJ, Rubin J, Frytak S. Failure of high-dose vitamin C (ascorbic acid) to benefit patients with advanced cancer: a controlled trail. N Engl J Med. 1979;301:687–90.
21. Moertel CG, Fleming TR, Creagan ET, Rubin J, O'Connell MJ, Aves MM. High-dose vitamin C versus placebo in the treatment of patients with advanced cancer who had no prior chemotherapy. N Engl J Med. 1985;312:137–41.
22. Richards E. The politics of therapeutic evaluation: the vitamin C and cancer controversy. J Nutr Med. 1994;4:215–46.
23. Blanchard J, Tozer TN, Rowland M. Pharmacokinetic perspective on megadosis of ascorbic acid. Am J Clin Nutr. 1997;66:1165–71.
24. Riordan NH, Riordan HD, Meng XL, Li Y, Jackson JA. Intravenous ascorbate as a tumor cytotoxic chemotherapeutic agent. Med Hypotheses. 1995;44:207–13.
25. Riordan NH, Riordan HD, Casciari JJ. Clinical and experimental experiences with intravenous vitamin C. J Orthomolec Med. 2000;15:201–13.
26. Schwartz J, Shklar G, Trickler D. Vitamin C enhances the development of carcinoma in the hamster buccal pouch experimental model. Oral Surg Oral Med Oral Pathol. 1993;76:718–22.
27. Shklar G, Schwartz J, Trickler D, Cheverie SR. The effectiveness of a mixture of beta carotene, alpha tocopherol, glutathione and ascorbic acid for cancer prevention. Nutr Cancer. 1993;20:145–51.
28. Cohen M, Bhagavan HN. Ascorbic acid and gastrointestinal cancer. J Am Coll Nutr. 1995;14:565–78.
29. Park CH. Vitamin C and leukemia and preleukemia cell growth. Prog Clin Biol Res. 1988;259:321–30.
30. Koh WS, Lee SJ, Lee H, Park C, Park MH, Kim WS, Yoon SS, Park K, Hong SI, Chung MH, Park CH. Differential effects and transport kinetics of ascorbate derivatives in leukemic cell lines. Anticancer Res. 1998;18:2487–93.
31. Prasad KN, Kumar R. Effect of Individual and multiple antioxidant vitamins on growth and morphology of human non-tumorigenic and tumorigenic parotid acinar cell in cultures. Nutr Cancer. 1996;26:11–9.
32. Hoffer LJ, Levine M, Assouline S, Melnychuk D, Padayatty SJ, Rosadiuk K, Rousseau C, Robitaille L, Miller WH Jr. Phase I clinical trial of iv ascorbic acid in advanced malignancy. Ann Oncol. 2008; 19(11):1969–74.

33. Riordan HD, Hunninghake RB, Riordan NH, Jackson JJ, Meng X, Taylor P, Casciari JJ, González MJ, Miranda-Massari JR, Mora EM, Rosario N, Rivera A. Intravenous ascorbic acid: protocol for its application and use. P R Health Sci J. 2003;22(3):287–90.
34. Stephenson CM, Levin RD, Spector T, Li CG. Phase I clinical trial to evaluate the safety, tolerability, and pharmacokinetics of high-dose intravenous ascorbic acid in patients with advanced cancer. Cancer Chemother Pharmacol. 2013;72:139–46.
35. Allwood MC, Kearney MC. Compatibility and stability of additives in parenteral nutrition admixtures. Nutrition. 1998;14(9):697–706.
36. Dupertuis YM, Morch A, Fathi M, Sierro C, Genton L, Kyle UG, Pichard C. Physical characteristics of total parenteral nutrition bags significantly affect the stability of vitamins C and B1: a controlled prospective study. JPEN J Parenter Enteral Nutr. 2002; 26(5):310–316.
37. Lavoie JC, Chessex P, Rouleau T, Migneault D, Comte B. Light-induced byproducts of vitamin C in multivitamin solutions. Clin Chem. 2004;50(1):135–40.
38. Levine M, Conry-Cantilena C, Wang Y, Welch RW, Washko PW, Dhariwal KR, Park JB, Lazarev A, Graumlich JF, King J, Cantilena LR. Vitamin C pharmacokinetics in healthy volunteers: evidence for a recommended dietary allowance. Proc Natl Acad Sci USA. 1996;93:3704–9.
39. Levine M, Wang Y, Padayatti SJ, Morrow J. A new recommended dietary allowance of vitamin C for healthy young women. Proc Natl Acad Sci USA. 2001;98(17):9842–6.
40. Graumlich JF, Ludden TM, Conry-Cantilena C, Cantilena LR Jr, Wang Y, Levine M. Pharmacokinetic model of ascorbic acid in healthy male volunteers during depletion and repletion. Pharm Res. 1997;14(9):1133–9.
41. Padayatty SJ, Sun H, Wang Y, Riordan HD, Hewitt SM, Katz A, Wesley RA, Levine M. Vitamin C pharmacokinetics: implications for oral and intravenous use. Ann Intern Med. 2004;140(7):533–7.
42. Casciari JJ, Riordan NH, Schmidt TL, Meng XL, Jackson JA, Riordan HD. Cytotoxicity of ascorbate, lipoic acid, and other antioxidants in hollow fibre in vitro tumours. Br J Cancer. 2001;84(11):1544–50.
43. Duconge J, Miranda-Massari JR, González MJ, Taylor PR, Riordan HD, Riordan NH, Casciari JJ, Alliston K. Vitamin C pharmacokinetics after continuous infusion in a patient with prostate cancer. Ann Pharmacother. 2007;41(6):1082–3.
44. Padayatty SJ, Levine M. Reevaluation of ascorbate in cancer treatment: emerging evidence, open minds and serendipity. J Am Coll Nutr. 2000;19(4):423–5.
45. Carr A, Frei B. Does vitamin C act as a pro-oxidant under physiological conditions? FASEB J. 1999;13:1007–24.
46. Chen Q, Espey MG, Krishna MC, Mitchell JB, Corpe CP, Buettner GR, Shacter E, Levine M. Pharmacologic ascorbic acid concentrations selectively kill cancer cells: action as a pro-drug to deliver hydrogen peroxide to tissues. Proc Natl Acad Sci USA. 2005;102(38):13604–9.
47. Frei B, Lawson S. Vitamin C and cancer revisited. Proc Natl Acad Sci USA. 2008;105 (32):11037–8.
48. Chen Q, Espey MG, Sun AY, Lee JH, Krishna MC, Shacter E, Choyke PL, Pooput C, Kirk KL, Buettner GR, Levine M. Ascorbate in pharmacologic concentrations selectively generates ascorbate radical and hydrogen peroxide in extracellular fluid in vivo. Proc Natl Acad Sci USA. 2007;104(21):8749–54.
49. Chen Q, Espey MG, Sun AY, Pooput C, Kirk KL, Krishna MC, Khosh DB, Drisko J, Levine M. Pharmacologic doses of ascorbate act as a prooxidant and decrease growth of aggressive tumor xenografts in mice. Proc Natl Acad Sci USA. 2008;105(32):11105–9.
50. Verrax J, Calderon PB. Pharmacologic concentrations of ascorbate are achieved by parenteral administration and exhibit antitumoral effects. Free Radic Biol Med. 2009;47(1):32–40.
51. Oberley TD, Oberley LW. Antioxidant enzyme levels in cancer. Histol Histopathol. 1997;12 (2):525–35.
52. Takemura Y, Satoh M, Satoh K, Hamada H, Sekido Y, Kubota S. High dose of ascorbic acid induces cell death in mesothelioma cells. Biochem Biophys Res Commun. 2010;394 (2):249–53.

53. Du J, Martin SM, Levine M, Wagner BA, Buettner GR, Wang SH, Taghiyev AF, Du C, Knudson CM, Cullen JJ. Mechanisms of ascorbate-induced cytotoxicity in pancreatic cancer. Clin Cancer Res. 2010;16(2):509–20.
54. Espey MG, Chen P, Chalmers B, Drisko J, Sun AY, Levine M, Chen Q. Pharmacologic ascorbate synergizes with gemcitabine in preclinical models of pancreatic cancer. Free Radic Biol Med. 2011;50(11):1610–9.
55. Belin S, Kaya F, Duisit G, Giacometti S, Ciccolini J, Fontés M. Antiproliferative effect of ascorbic acid is associated with the inhibition of genes necessary to cell cycle progression. PLoS One. 2009;4(2):e4409.
56. Yeom CH, Lee G, Park JH, Yu J, Park S, Yi SY, Lee HR, Hong YS, Yang J, Lee S. High dose concentration administration of ascorbic acid inhibits tumor growth in BALB/C mice implanted with sarcoma 180 cancer cells via the restriction of angiogenesis. J Transl Med. 2009;11(7):70.
57. Pollard HB, Levine MA, Eidelman O, Pollard M. Pharmacological ascorbic acid suppresses syngeneic tumor growth and metastases in hormone-refractory prostate cancer. In Vivo. 2010; 24(3):249–255.
58. Padayatty SJ, Sun AY, Chen Q, Espey MG, Drisko J, Levine M. Vitamin C: intravenous use by complementary and alternative medicine practitioners and adverse effects. PLoS One. 2010;5(7):e11414.
59. Riordan HD, Casciari JJ, González MJ, Riordan NH, Miranda-Massari JR, Taylor P, Jackson JA. A pilot clinical study of continuous intravenous ascorbate in terminal cancer patients. P R Health Sci J. 2005;24(4):269–76.
60. Campbell GD Jr, Steinberg MH, Bower JD. Letter: ascorbic acid-induced hemolysis in G-6-PD deficiency. Ann Intern Med. 1975;82(6):810.
61. Rees DC, Kelsey H, Richards JD. Acute haemolysis induced by high dose ascorbic acid in glucose-6-phosphate dehydrogenase deficiency. BMJ. 1993;306(6881):841–2.
62. Campbell A, Jack T. Acute reactions to mega ascorbic acid therapy in malignant disease. Scott Med J. 1979;24(2):151–3.
63. McAllister CJ, Scowden EB, Dewberry FL, Richman A. Renal failure secondary to massive infusion of vitamin C. JAMA. 1984;252(13):1684.
64. Lawton JM, Conway LT, Crosson JT, Smith CL, Abraham PA. Acute oxalate nephropathy after massive ascorbic acid administration. Arch Intern Med. 1985;145(5):950–1.
65. Robitaille L, Mamer OA, Miller WH Jr, Levine M, Assouline S, Melnychuk D, Rousseau C, Hoffer LJ. Oxalic acid excretion after intravenous ascorbic acid administration. Metabolism. 2009;58(2):263–9.
66. Heinz-Schmidt K, Hagmaier V, Hornig DH, Vuilleumier JP, Rutishauser G. Urinary oxalate excretion after large intakes of ascorbic acid in man. Am J Clin Nat. 1981;34:305–11.
67. Sutton JL, Basu TK, Dickerson JWT. Effect of large doses of ascorbic acid in man on some nitrogenous components of urine. Human Nutr. 1983;37A:136–40.
68. Erden F, Hacisalihoglu A, Kocer Z, Simsek B, Nebioglu S. Effects of vitamin C intake on whole blood plasma, leukocyte and urine ascorbic acid and urine oxalic acid levels. Acta Vitaminol Enzymol. 1985;7:123–30.
69. Tsao CS, Leung PY. Urinary ascorbic acid levels following the withdrawal of large doses of ascorbic acid in guinea pigs. J Nutr. 1988;118:895–900.
70. Gerster H. No contribution of ascorbic acid to renal calcium oxalate stones. Ann Nutr Metab. 1997;41:269–82.
71. Wandzilak TR, D'Andre SD, Davis PA, Williams HE. Effect of high dose vitamin C on urinary oxalate levels. J Urol. 1994;151:834–7.
72. Barness LA. Safety consideration with high ascorbic acid dosage. Ann NY Acad Sci. 1974;258:253–8.
73. Carthcart RF. Vitamin C tritrating to bowel tolerance, anascorbemia and acute induced scurvy. Med Hypotheses. 1981;7:1359–76.
74. Carthcart RF. The method of determining proper doses of vitamin C for the treatment of diseases by titrating to bowel intolerance. Austral Nurses J. 1981;9:9–13.

75. González MJ. Ascorbic acid and selenium interaction: its relevance in carcinogenesis. J Ortomolec Med. 1990;5:67–9.
76. Riordan NH, Riordan HD, Meng XL, Li Y, Jackson JA. Intravenous ascorbate as a tumor cytotoxic chemotherapeutic agent. Med Hypotheses. 1995;44:207–13.
77. Riordan HD, Jackson JA, Schultz M. Case study: high-dose intravenous vitamin C in the treatment of a patient with adenocarcinoma of the kidney. J Orthomolec Med. 1990;5:5–7.
78. Jackson JA, Riordan HD, Hunninghake RE, Riordan NH. High dose intravenous Vitamin C and long time survival of a patient with cancer of the head of the pancreas. J Orthomolec Med. 1995;10:87–8.
79. Riordan NH, Riordan HD, Casciari JJ. Clinical and experimental experiences with intravenous vitamin C. J Orthomolec Med. 2000;15:201–13.
80. Klenner FR. Observations on the dose and administration of ascorbic acid when employed beyond the range of a vitamin in human pathology. J Apl Nutr. 1971;23:61–88.
81. Cathcart RF. Vitamin C; the non-toxic, non-rate-limited antioxidant free radical scavenger. Med Hypotheses. 1985;18:61–77.

Chapter 2
Anticancer Mechanisms of Vitamin C

Cancer Preventative Mechanisms of Vitamin C

Antioxidant Properties of Vitamin C

Vitamin C is considered a very strong reductant and radical scavenger. Vitamin C reduces unstable oxygen, nitrogen, and sulfur radicals. In addition, it acts as primary defense against aqueous radicals in blood [1, 2]. In studies with human plasma, vitamin C protected plasma lipids against peroxidative damage induced by aqueous peroxyl radicals [3]. Thus, by efficiently trapping peroxyl radicals in the aqueous phase before they can reach the lipid-rich membranes and initiate lipid peroxidation, vitamin C can protect bio-membranes against primary peroxidative damage. Vitamin C may also protect membranes against lipid peroxidation due to its synergistic antioxidant function with vitamin E. Vitamin C may enhance or reinstate the activity of tocopherol (vitamin E), the principal lipid soluble antioxidant [1]. Vitamin C reacts with the tocopheroxyl (chromanoxyl) radical that arises in cell membranes as a result of vitamin E antioxidant activity; and simultaneously regenerates tocopherol and transfers the oxidative challenge to the aqueous phase [3]. At this point, the less reactive ascorbate radical can be enzymatically reduced back to ascorbic acid by an NADH-dependent system [4–6]. This probably explains how ascorbate reduces nitrates and prevents the formation of carcinogenic nitrosamines [7]. Vitamin C is found naturally in the following foods: broccoli, cabbage, potatoes, peas, red peppers, brussel sprouts, kale, cauliflower, cantaloupe, strawberries, mangoes, tangerines, orange, grapefruit, lemons, and limes.

© The Author(s) 2014
M.J. Gonzalez and J.R. Miranda-Massari, *New Insights on Vitamin C and Cancer*,
SpringerBriefs in Cancer Research, DOI 10.1007/978-1-4939-1890-4_2

Primary Anticancer Mechanisms of Vitamin C

Oxidative, Oxidant, and Pro-oxidant Properties of Vitamin C

Vitamin C not only possesses antioxidant activity, but also can generate cytotoxic activity at higher concentrations [8–10]. It has also been suggested that vitamin C may promote oxidative metabolism by inhibiting the utilization of pyruvate for anaerobic glycolysis [11]. Vitamin C in high concentrations inhibits prostaglandins of the 2-series (arachidonic acid derived), which have been correlated with inflammation and increased cell proliferation [12]. A growth inhibitory action has been reported for vitamin C or its derivatives in at least seven types of tumor cells [13–19]. This inhibitory activity was not observed in normal fibroblasts [13–18], while other researchers have reported a fibroblast inhibition [19–23]. Nevertheless, all reports concur that this cytotoxic effect produced by vitamin C in an array of cell lines (mostly malignant) has been associated with its pro-oxidant activity [8, 24–30]. Vitamin C and its radical potentiate the activation of transcription factor NF-kappa B, which has been associated with inhibition of cell growth [31].

Hydrogen Peroxide and Vitamin C

Vitamin C can generate hydrogen peroxide (a reactive oxygen species) upon oxidation (with oxygen) in biological systems [32–34]. This action can be enhanced by divalent cations such as iron and copper [10, 24, 35]. Hydrogen peroxide may further generate additional reactive species, such as the hydroxyl radical and secondary products of oxidation, such as aldehydes. These reactive species can compromise cell viability mainly by damaging the cell membranes and mitochondria. Malignant cells are relatively deficient in catalase activity [27, 35–40]. However, these oxidative reactions may only form in minute quantities in healthy organisms. This is mainly because most transition metal ions are bound to proteins in serum, which makes them unavailable to participate in biochemical reactions [41]. Nevertheless, these oxidation reactions may take place in pathological states such as malignancy, in which cohesive forces that inhibit the liberation of the metal ion from the proteins as well as the control of the cell's replication mechanisms are drastically reduced [41]. These reactive species are capable of inducing multiple negative cellular effects such as DNA strand breaks, disruption of membrane function via lipid peroxidation, and depletion of cellular ATP [39]. The failure to maintain high ATP production (cell energy level) may be a consequence of oxidative inactivation of key enzymes, especially those related to the Krebs cycle and the electron transport system. A distorted mitochondrial function (transmembrane potential) may result. This aspect could be suggestive of an important mitochondrial involvement in the carcinogenic process [42]. In this respect, vitamin C may serve yet another metabolic and physiological function by providing reductive energy, i.

e., the electrons necessary to direct energy pathways in the mitochondria [43–47]. Interestingly, vitamin C has been detected within the mitochondria where it is also regenerated [48].

In general, the cytotoxicity induced by vitamin C seems to be primarily mediated by hydrogen peroxide [13–16, 21, 36, 49–51]. Of interest, is the observation that in proliferating cells very low levels of hydrogen peroxide (3–15 μM) stimulate cell division, whereas greater concentrations induce cell growth arrest, apoptosis and/or necrosis [50]. It has also been shown that the amount of hydrogen peroxide generated by the cells was proportionally dependent on the vitamin C concentration and inhibited by serum [20, 51–53]. Human serum, as part of its normal contents, has certain proteins such as albumin and glutathione with antioxidant capacity that may stabilize vitamin C (directly or indirectly by chelating available transition metals). In addition, serum contains antioxidant enzymes such as catalase, which decomposes hydrogen peroxide. Other antioxidant enzymes including glutathione peroxidase and superoxide dismutase complement the catalase enzymatic function.

Hydrogen peroxide is most likely generated during ascorbate's metabolic oxidation to dehydroascorbate. Hydrogen peroxide reduces cellular levels of thiols and can initiate membrane lipid peroxidation [13–19, 35–37, 49, 54–56]. As previously mentioned, the antiproliferative action of vitamin C in malignant cultured cells, animal, and human tumor xenografts has been augmented by the addition of the cupric ion, a catalyst for the oxidation of vitamin C [19, 24–26, 57–59]. In addition, the combination of vitamin C and copper has been shown to inactivate lactate dehydrogenase [60], the enzyme responsible for the reduction of pyruvate to lactate (a metabolic dead end product prevalent in anaerobic environments such as in cancer). Copper in the form of copper sulfate may also inhibit tyrosinase activity [61, 62]. It has also been suggested that the selective toxicity of vitamin C in malignant cells may be due to reduced levels of antioxidant enzymes, catalase, superoxide dismutase, and glutathione peroxidase [63] in these cells, leading to cellular damage through the accumulation of hydrogen peroxide [29, 57, 64–68]. There is a 10- to 100-fold greater content of catalase in normal cells than in tumor cells [29, 64].

Furthermore, the addition of vitamin K3 (menadione) to vitamin C produces a synergistic antitumor activity [69–73]. Since menadione is reduced intracellularly via one or two electron transfer action (probably by vitamin C), this may lead to formation of hydrogen peroxide and other reactive oxygen species, concomitant with the depletion of glutathione. Decreases of glutathione have also been associated with vitamin C metabolism [74]. Interestingly, a new form of cell death (autoschizis) has been described for this synergistic vitamin (vitamins C and K) phenomenon in which tumor cells undergo profound perturbations of cytoskeleton and membranes that ultimately kill the cells by a form of cell death that is distinct from apoptosis, oncosis, or necrosis [71–75]. For this reason, the combination of megadoses of IV ascorbate together with oxygen, vitamin K, lipoic acid, carnitine, magnesium, Coenzyme Q10, and small doses of copper may seem logical as part of a non-toxic treatment protocol for cancer. Intravenous administration of vitamin C can yield very high plasma levels that seem to be necessary for vitamin C's toxic effect on malignant cells [76–79].

Other Vitamin C Oxidation Products with Anti-cancer Potential

Furthermore, vitamin C oxidation products such as dehydroascorbic acid, 2,3-diketogulonic acid, and 5-methyl 1-3,4-dehydroxytetrone, all degradation products of ascorbic acid, have demonstrated antitumor activity [19, 24–27]. In addition, other compounds arising from the oxidation or degradation of ascorbate can inhibit tumor growth. The most effective ones are: gamma-cronolactone and 3-hydroxy-2-pyrone. The available evidence suggests that these vitamin C oxidation products and/or metabolic by-products have a function in controlling mitotic activity. All active compounds consist of an unsaturated lactose ring with a double bond conjugated with a carbonyl group, suggesting that this particular structural feature of the lactose ring may be relevant in the antitumor activity [19]. The antitumor activity shown by these compounds could be due to their ability to produce active molecular species that inhibit tumor growth such as hydrogen peroxide and certain aldehydes. Most of these compounds are very unstable and their growth inhibitory activities could be attributed to their chemical instability which favors the formation of reactive species. These antiproliferative mechanisms of vitamin C and/or its oxidation products on tumor cells are probably of a very complex nature, since they seem to involve a series of pleiotropic chain reactions.

Large amounts of vitamin C intake can change the levels of certain amino acids in body fluids [80–83] and may deplete the bioavailability of lysine, glutamine and cysteine, two amino acids which are required for rapidly growing tumors [84]. Experiments using tissue homogenate show that the interactions between vitamin C, metal ions, and oxygen are capable of inducing structural changes in protein [82–84]. These electron transfer reactions need a conductor in order to proceed; and proteins can serve as electron conductors for these reactions. Metal ions, such as copper, are good electron conductors because their valence bonds are partially filled. The resulting molecules contain one or more uncoupled electrons and are very reactive-free radicals.

Dehydroascorbic acid (the oxidized, nonionic, and more lipid soluble form of ascorbate) and the semi-dehydroascorbic acid radical have been shown to promote lipid peroxidation [19]. One of us (MJG) has demonstrated that secondary products of lipid peroxidation have an inhibitory action on human malignant cell proliferation [38, 40, 49, 54]. There is evidence to suggest that dehydroascorbic acid may work as a mitotic inhibitor in vivo [76]. Dehydroascorbic acid may prevent cell division by inhibiting protein synthesis at the ribosomal level [76]. Interestingly, prolonged exposure to high concentrations of dehydroascorbic acid may cause irreparable damage resulting ultimately in complete lysis of the cells [76].

In summary, there are various oxidative species related to vitamin C biophysiology that may produce a cytostatic or cytotoxic action. Moreover, a synergistic interaction seems very likely involving these cell growth inhibitory mechanisms.

Secondary Anticancer Mechanisms of Vitamin C: Host Resistance to Cancer

Vitamin C and Intracellular Matrix

Vitamin C metabolism is associated with other mechanisms known to be involved in host resistance to malignant disease. Cancer patients are significantly depleted of vitamin C. This could indicate an increase requirement and utilization of this substance to potentiate these various resistance mechanisms. Scurvy results from the severe dietary lack of vitamin C. It is a syndrome of generalized tissue disintegration at all levels, involving the dissolution of intercellular ground substance, the disruption of collagen bundles, and the lysis of the inter-epithelial and inter-endothelial cement. This disintegration leads to ulceration with secondary bacterial colonization, to vascular disorganization with edema and interstitial hemorrhage, and to generalized undifferentiated cellular proliferation throughout the tissue reverting to a primitive form [85]. The generalized stromal changes of scurvy are identical to the local stromal changes observed in the immediate vicinity of invading neoplastic cells [86]. Thus, stomal resistance may be a physical line of defense against cancer by encapsulating neoplastic cells with a dense fibrous tissue. This feature can be enhanced by high doses of vitamin C. Vitamin C also enhances the resistance of the intercellular ground substance to local infiltration.

A brisk lymphocytic response is a systemic factor indicative of enhanced host resistance and is associated with a more favorable prognosis of the disease. In order to proliferate, cells must escape the restraint imposed by highly viscous intercellular glycosaminoglycans and can do this by the release of the enzyme hyaluronidase [87]. There is evidence that a physiological hyaluronidase inhibitor is an oligo-glycosaminoglycan that requires ascorbic acid for its synthesis [88]. Decreases in hyaluronic acid have been shown to be conducive to cell proliferation [89]. In addition, ascorbate is involved in the synthesis of collagen. Collagen rich extracellular matrix including the basement membrane is a major barrier to the metastatic and invasive spread of cancer cells [85]. The intercellular matrix is reinforced by a tri-dimensional network of interlacing collagen fibers. The amount of collagen present determines the strength of the tissue and also its resistance to malignant infiltration. Lack of ascorbate sharply reduces hydroxylation of prolyl and lysyl residues into hydroxyproline and hydroxylysine, leading to instability of the triple helix of collagen [90], which is a common feature in scurvy and also present in cancer. This is also of importance in vitamin C's role on wound healing including decubital ulcers, surgery recovery, and other traumatic injuries [91].

Vitamin C and Immuno-competence

Ascorbate is essential to ensure the efficient working of the immune system. The immuno-competence mechanisms are a combination of humoral and cell-mediated defensive reactions with ascorbate involved in a number of ways. In terms of humoral immuno-competence, ascorbate is essential for immunoglobulin synthesis [92]. In cell-mediated immunity, immuno-competence is exercised overwhelmingly by lymphocytes which contain high concentrations of ascorbate relative to other cells. In addition, ascorbate is required for active phagocytosis [93]. Ascorbate has also been shown to enhance interferon production [93–95].

Ascorbic acid has other identified functions related to cancer prevention. Ascorbate is required by the mixed function oxidases for the hydroxylation of amino acids [85]. The mixed function oxidases are a group of closely related microsomal enzymes that metabolize many classes of compounds and are particularly important in the inactivation of chemical carcinogens. Microsomal metabolism of carcinogens yields products generally more water soluble which greatly increases their rate of excretion. In addition, ascorbate has been shown to protect against nitrate-induced carcinogenesis [96]. Another important anticancer function of vitamin C when provided in large quantities is that it enhances the removal of sodium via the urine thereby reducing the level of sodium ions in the serum. In cancer, there is a disturbed sodium/potassium ratio. It has been suggested that vitamin C may also have a role inhibiting prostaglandins of the two series in carcinoma cells [97, 98]. In the process of prostaglandin biosynthesis, the release of arachidonic acid from cell membrane phospholipids is implicated as one of the synergistic signals leading to cell proliferation. Also, vitamin C has been shown to stabilize p53, a protein involved in cell proliferation control [99, 100].

References

1. Niki E. Action of ascorbic acid as a scavenger of active and stable oxygen radicals. Am J Clin Nutr. 1991;54:1119s–24s.
2. Frei B, England L, Ames B. Ascorbate is an outstanding antioxidant in human blood plasma. Proc Natl Acad Sci USA. 1989;86:6377–81.
3. Vandenberg JJ, Kuypers FA, Roelofsen B. Op den Kamp JA. The cooperative action of vitamins E and C in the protection against peroxidation of parinanic acid in human erythrocyte menbranes. Chem Phys Lipids. 1990;53:309–20.
4. Chan A. Partners in defense: vitamin E and vitamin C. Can J Physiol Pharmacol. 1993;71:725–31.
5. Levine M, Dhariwal K, Washko PW, Butler JD, Welch RN, Wang YH, Bergslen P. Ascorbic acid and in situ kinetics: a new approach to vitamin requirements. Am J Clin Nutr. 1991;54:1157s–62s.
6. Packer J, Slater T, Wilson R. Direct observation of a free radical interaction between vitamin E and vitamin C. Nature. 1979;278:737–8.

7. Burton GW, Wronska U, Stone L. Biokinetics of dietary RRR-OC-tocopherol in the male guinea pig at three dietary levels of vitamin C does not spare vitamin E in vivo. Lipids. 1990;25:199–210.

8. González MJ, Mora E, Riordan NH, Riordan HD, Mojica P. Rethinking vitamin C and cancer: an update on nutritional oncology. Cancer Prev Intl. 1998;3:215–24.

9. Yamamoto K, Takahashi M, Niki E. Role of iron and ascorbic acid in the oxidation of methyl linoleate micelles. Chem Lett. 1987;1:49–52.

10. Rowly DA, Halliwell B. Superoxide-dependents and ascorbate-dependent formation of hydroxy radicals in the presence of copper salts: a physiologically significant reaction? Arch Biochem Biophys. 1983;225:279–84.

11. Ramp WK, Thorton PA. The effects of ascorbic acid on the glycolytic and respiratory metabolism of embryonic chick tibias. Cal Tissue Res. 1968;2:77–82.

12. Beetens JR, Hermen AG. Ascorbic acid and Prostaglandin formation. Int J Vitam Nutr Res. 1983;24(Suppl):131s–44s.

13. Mikino Y, Sakagami H, Takeda M. Induction of cell death by ascorbic acid derivatives in human renal carcinoma and glyobastoma cell lines. Anticancer Res. 1999;19:3125–32.

14. Nakamura Y, Yamafuji K. Antitumor activities of oxidized products of ascorbic acid. Sci Bull Fac Kyushu Univ. 1968;23:119–25.

15. Yamafuji K, Nakamura Y, Omura H, Soeda T, Gyotoku K. Antitumor potency of ascorbic, dehydroascorbic or 2,3-diketogulonic acid and their action on deoxyribonucleic acid. Z Krebsforsh Klin Onkol Cancer Res Clin Oncol. 1971;76:1–7.

16. Omura H, Tomita Y, Yasuhiko N. Antitumor potentiality of some ascorbate derivaties. J Fac Agr Kyushu Univ. 1974;18:181–9.

17. Tomita Y, Eto M, Lio M. Antitumor potency of 3-methyl-3,4-dihydroxytetrone. Sci Bull Fac Agr Kyushu Univ. 1974;28:131–7.

18. Poydock ME, Reikert D, Rice J, Aleandri L. Inhibiting effect of dehydroascorbic acid on cell division in ascites tumors in mice. Exp Cell Biol. 1982;50:34–8.

19. Leung PY, Miyashita K, Young M, Tsao CS. Cytotoxic effect of ascorbate and its derivative on cultured malignant and non malignant cell lines. Anticancer Res. 1993;13:47–80.

20. Avakawa N, Nemoto S, Suzuki E, Otsuka M. Role of hydrogen peroxide in the inhibitory effect os ascorbate on cell growth. J Nutr Sci Vitaminol. 1994;40:219–27.

21. Peterkofsky B, Prather W. Cytotoxicity of ascorbate and other reducing agents towards cultured fibroblasts as a result of hydrogen peroxide formation. J Cell Physiol. 1971;90:61–70.

22. Yve B, Niedra JT, Baum JL. Effects of ascorbic acid on cultured rabbit endothelial cells. Invest Opthal Mol Vis Sci. 1980;19:1471–6.

23. Jampel HD. Ascorbic acid is cytotoxic to dividing human Tenon's capsule fibroblasts. Arch Opthal Mol. 1990;108:1323–5.

24. Tsao CS, Dunhan WB, Leung PY. In vivo antineoplastic activity of ascorbic acid for human mammary tumor. In vivo. 1988;2:147–50.

25. Tsao CS, Dunhan WB, Leung PY. Effect of ascorbic acid and its derivatives on the growth of human mammary tumor xenografts in mice. Cancer J. 1989;5:53–9.

26. Poydock ME. Effect of combined ascorbic acid and B12 on survival of mice implanted with Erlich carcinoma and L1210 leukemia. Am Clin Nutr. 1982;54:1261s–5s.

27. Edgar JA. Dehydroascorbic acid and cell division. Nature. 1970;227:24–6.

28. Bram S, Froussard P, Guichard M, Jasmine C, Augery Y, Sinoussi-barre F, Wray W. Vitamin C preferential toxicity for malignant melanoma cells. Nature. 1980;284:629–31.

29. Riordan NH, Riordan HD, Meng XL, Li Y, Jackson JA. Intravenous ascorbate as a tumor cytotoxic chemotherapeutic agent. Med Hypotheses. 1995;44:207–13.

30. Sakagami H, Satoh K. Pro-oxidant action of two antioxidants: ascorbic acid and gallic acid. Anticancer Res. 1997;17:221–4.

31. Muñoz E, Blazquez MV, Ortiz C, Gómez-Díaz C, Navas P. Role of ascorbate in the activation of NF-κB by tumour necrosis factor-α in T-cells. Biochem J. 1997;325:23–8.

32. Halliwell B. Vitamin C: antioxidant or pro-oxidant in vivo? Free Red Res. 1996;25:439–54.

33. Alcain FJ, Buron MI. Ascorbate on cell growth and differentiation. J Bioenerg Biomembr. 1996;26:393–8.
34. Asano K, Satoh K, Hosaka M, Arakawa N, Wagaki M, Hisamitsu T, Maeda M, Kochi M, Sakagami H. Production of hydrogen peroxide in cancerous tissue by intravenous administration of sodium 5,6 benzylidene-L-ascorbate. Anticancer Res. 1999;19:229–36.
35. Jonas SK, Riley PA, Willson RL. Hydrogen peroxide cytotoxicity. Biochem J. 1989;264:651–5.
36. Clement MV, Ramalingam J, Long LH, Halliwell B. The in vivo cytotoxicity of ascorbate depends on the culture medium used to perform assay and involves hydrogen peroxide. Antiox Redox Signal. 2001;3:157–63.
37. Sakagami H, Satoh K, Kochi M. Comparative study of the antitumor action between sodium 5,6 benzylidene-L-ascorbate and sodium ascorbate. Anticancer Res. 1997;17:4401–52.
38. González MJ, Schemel RA, Gray JI, Dugan LJR, Sheffield LG, Welsch CW. Effect of dietary fat growth of MCF-7 and MDA-MB231 human breast carcinomas in athymic nude mice: relationship between carcinoma growth and lipid peroxidation products level. Carcinogenesis. 1991;12:1231–5.
39. González MJ. Lipid peroxidation and tumor growth: an inverse relationship. Med Hypotheses. 1992;38:106–10.
40. González MJ, Riordan NH. The paradoxical role of lipid peroxidation on carcinogenesis and tumor growth. Med Hypotheses. 1996;46:503–4.
41. Gutteridge JMC, Richmond R, Halliwell B. Oxygen free-radicals and lipid peroxidation: inhibition by the protein caeruloplasmin. FEBS Lett. 1980;112:269–72.
42. Gonzalez MJ, Miranda-Massari JR, Duconge J, Riordan NH, Ichim T, Quintero-Del-Rio AI, Ortiz N. The bioenergetic theory of carcinogenesis. Med Hypotheses. 2012;79:433–9.
43. Szent-Gyorgyi A. The living state and cancer. Physiol Chem Physics. 1980;12:99–110.
44. Schwarz JL. The dual roles of nutrients as antioxidants and pro-oxidants: their effects on tumor cell growth. J Nutr. 1996;126:1221S–7S.
45. Sigal A, King CG. The relationship of vitamin C to glucose tolerance in the guinea pig. J Biol Chem. 1936;166:489–92.
46. Landauver W, Sopher D. Succinate, glycerophosphate and ascorbate as sources of cellular energy as antiteratogens. J Embryol Exp Morph. 1970;24:187–202.
47. Cathcart RF. A unique function for ascorbate. Med Hypotheses. 1991;35:32–7.
48. Li Y, Cobb CE, Hill KE, Burk RF, May JM. Mitochondrial uptake and recycling of ascorbic acid. Arch Biochem Biophys. 2001;387:143–53.
49. González MJ, Schemmel RA, Dugan L Jr, Gray JI, Welsch CW. Dietary fish oil inhibits human breast carcinoma growth: a function of increased lipid peroxidation. Lipids. 1993;28:827–32.
50. Sakagami H, Satoh K, Hakeda Y, Kumegawa M. Apoptosis-inducing activity of vitamin C and vitamin K. Cell Molec Biol. 2000;46:129–43.
51. Iwasaka K, Koyama N, Nogaki A, Murayama S, Tamura A, Takano H, Takahama M, Kochi M, Satoh K, Sakagami H. Role of hydrogen peroxide in cytotoxicity induction by ascorbates and other redox compounds. Anticancer Res. 1998;18:4333–7.
52. Davies KJA. The broad spectrum of responses to oxidants in proliferating cells: a new paradigm for oxidative stress. Life Sci. 1999;48:41–7.
53. Dasgupta A, Zdunek T. In vitro lipid peroxidation of human serum catalyzed by cupric ion: antioxidant rather than pro-oxidant role of ascorbate. Life Sci. 1992;50:875–82.
54. Sakagami H, Satoh K, Sugaya K, Iida M, Hirota N, Matsumoto K, Kimura S, Gomi K, Taguchi S, Kato S, Takeda M. Effect of the type of serum in the medium on sodium ascorbate-induced toxicity. Anticancer Res. 1996;16:1937–42.
55. Sakagami H, Satoh K, Taguchi S, Takeda M. Inhibition of cytotoxic activity of ascorbate by human cancer patient sera. Anticancer Res. 1997;17:425–8.
56. González MJ. Fish oil, lipid peroxidation and mammary tumor growth. J Am Coll Nutr. 1995;14:325–35.

57. Iyanagi T, Yamazaki I, Anan KF. One electron oxidation-reduction properties of ascorbic acid. Biochem Acta. 1985;806:255–61.
58. Venugopal M, Jamison JM, Gilloteaux J, Koch JA, Summers M, Giammar D, Sowich C, Summers JL. Synergistic antitumor activity of vitamins C and K 3 on human urologic tumor cell lines. Life Sci. 1996;59:1389–400.
59. Satoh K, Kadofuku T, Sakagami H. Copper but not iron, enhances apoptosis-inducing activity of antioxidants. Anticancer Res. 1997;17:2487–90.
60. González MJ, Miranda-Massari JR, Mora EM, Jiménez IZ, Matos MI, Riordan HD, Casciari JJ, Riordan NH, Rodríguez M, Guzmán A. Orthomolecular oncology: a mechanic view intravenous ascorbate's chemotherapeutic activity. PR Health Sci J. 2002;21:39–41.
61. González MJ, Mora EM, Miranda-Massari JR, Matta J, Riordan HD, Riordan NH. Inhibition of human breast carcinoma cell proliferation by ascorbate and copper. PR Health Sci J. 2002;21:21–30.
62. Nelson SR, Pazdernik TL, Samson FE. Copper plus ascorbate inactivates lactate dehydrogenase. Are oxygen radicals involved? Proc West Pharmacol Soc. 1992;35:37–41.
63. Powers HJ, Gibson AT, Bates CJ, Primhak RA, Beresford J. Does vitamin C intake influence the rate of tyrosine catabolism in premature babies? Ann Nutr Metab. 1994;38:166–73.
64. Palumbo A, Misuraca G, D'Ischia M, Prota G. Effect of metal ions on the kinetics of tyrosine oxidation catalysed by tyrosinase. Biochem J. 1985;288:647–51.
65. Sun Y, Oberley LW, Oberley TD, Elwell JH, Sierra-Rivera E. Lowered antioxidant enzymes in spontaneously transformed embryonic mouse liver cells in culture. Carcinogenesis. 1993;14:1437–46.
66. Benade L, Howard T, Burk D. Synergistic killing of Ehrlich ascites carcinoma cells by ascorbate and 3-amino-1,2,4,-triazole. Oncology. 1969;23:33–43.
67. Punnonen K, Ahotupa M, Asaishi K, Hyoty M, Kudo R, Punnonen R. Antioxidant enzyme activities and oxidative stress in human breast cancer. J Cancer Res Clin Oncol. 1994;120:374–7.
68. Jaruga P, Olinste R. Activity of antioxidant enzymes in cancer diseases. Postepy Hig Med Dosw. 1994;48:443–55.
69. Sestili P, Brandi G, Brambilla L, Cattabeni F, Cantoni O. Hydrogen peroxide mediates the killing of U937 tumor cells elicited by pharmacologically attainable concentrations of ascorbic acid cell death prevention by extracellular catalase from cultured erythrocytes of fibroblasts. J Pharmacol Exp Therapeutics. 1996;277:1719–25.
70. Sun Y, Colburn NH, Oberley LW. Depression of catalase gene expression after inmortalization and transformation of mouse liver cells. Carcinogenesis. 1993;14:1505–10.
71. Bozzi A, Mavelli I, Mondovi B, Strom R, Rotilio G. Differential sensitivity of tumor cells to externally generated hydrogen peroxide: role of glutathione and related enzymes. Cancer Biochem Biophys. 1979;3:135–41.
72. Noto V, Taper HS, Jiang YH, Janssens J, Bonte J, De Loeker W. Effects of sodium ascorbate (vitamin C) and 2-methyl-1,4 naphthoquinone (vitamin K 3) treatment of human tumor cell growth in vitro. Cancer. 1989;63:901–6.
73. Gilloteaux J, Jamison JM, Arnold D, Ervin E, Echroat L, Docherty JJ, Neal D, Summers JL. Cancer cell necrosis by autoshizis: synergism of antitumor activity of vitamin C: vitamin K 3 on human bladder carcinoma T-24 cells. Scanning. 1998;20:564–75.
74. Gilloteaux J, Jamison JM, Ervin E, Arnold D, Summers JL. Scanning electron microscopy and transmission electron microscopy aspects of the synergistic antitumor activity of vitamin C/vitamin K 3 combinations against human T-24 bladder carcinoma: another kind of cell death. Scanning. 1998;20:208–9.
75. Gilloteaux J, Jamison JM, Arnold D, Taper HS, Summers JL. Ultrastructural aspects of autoshizis: a new cancer cell death induced by the synergistic action of ascorbate/menadione on human bladder carcinoma cells. Ultrastruct Pathol. 2001;25:183–92.
76. Grad JM, Bahlis NJ, Reis I, Oshiro MM, Dalton WS, Boise LH. Ascorbic acid enhances arsenic trioxide-induced cytotoxicity in multiple myeloma cells. Blood. 2001;98:805–13.

77. Jamison JM, Gilloteaux J, Taper HS, Calderón PB, Summers JL. Autoshizis: a novel cell death. Biochemical Pharmacol. 2002;63:1773–83.
78. Riordan HD, Jackson JA, Schultz M. Case study: high-dose intravenous vitamin C in the treatment of a patient with adenocarcinoma of the kidney. J Orthomolec Med. 1990;5:5–7.
79. Jackson JA, Riordan HD, Hunninghake RE, Riordan NH. High dose intravenous vitamin C and long time survival of a patient with cancer of the head of the pancreas. J Orthomolec Med. 1995;10:87–8.
80. Riordan NH, Riordan HD, Casciari JJ. Clinical and experimental experiences with intravenous vitamin C. J Orthomolec Med. 2000;15:201–13.
81. Casciari JJ, Riordan NH, Schmidt TL, Meng XL, Jackson JA, Riordan HD. Cytotoxicity of ascorbate, lipoic acid and other antioxidants in hollow fiber in vitro tumours. Brit J Cancer. 2001;84:1544–50.
82. Lykkesfeldt J, Hagen TM, Vinarsky V, Ames BN. Age associated decline in ascorbic acid concentration, recycling and biosynthesis in rat hepatocytes-reversal with (R)-α-lipoic acid supplementation. FASEB J. 1998;12:1183–9.
83. Tsao CS, Miyashita K. Effects of high intake of ascorbic acid on plasma levels of amino acids. IRCS Med Sci. 1984;12:1052–3.
84. Tsao CS, Miyashita K. Effects of large intake of ascorbic acid on the urinary excretion of amino acids and related compounds. IRCS Med Sci. 1985;13:855–6.
85. Cameron E, Pauling L, Leibovitz B. Ascorbic acid and cancer: a review. Cancer Res. 1979;39:663–81.
86. McCormick WJ. Cancer: a collagen disease, secondary to a nutritional deficiency? Arch Pediatr. 1959;76:166–71.
87. Dresden MH, Heilman SA, Schmidt JD. Collagenolytic enzymes in human neoplasms. Cancer Res. 1972;32:993–6.
88. Cameron E, Pauling L. Ascorbic acid and the glycosaminoglycan: an orthomolecular approach to cancer and other diseases. Oncology. 1973;27:181–92.
89. Yoneda M, Shimizu S, Nishi Y, Yamagata M, Suzuki S, Kimata K. Hyaluronic acid dependent change in the extracellular matrix of mouse dermal fibroblasts that is conductive to cell proliferation. J Cell Sci. 1998;90:275–86.
90. Kennedy JF. Chemical and biochemical aspects of the glycosaminoglycans and proteoglycans in health and disease. Adv Clin Chem. 1976;18:1–101.
91. Ringsdorf WM Jr, Cheraskin E. Vitamin C and human wound healing. Oral Surg. 1982;53:231–6.
92. Lewin S, Vitamin C. Its molecular biology and medical potential. NY: Academic Press; 1976.
93. Goetzl EJ, Wasserman SI, Gigli I, Austen KF. Enhancement of random migration and chemotactic response of human leukocytes by ascorbic acid. J Clin Invest. 1974;53:813–8.
94. Siegel BV. Enhancement of interferon production by poly (r1), poly (rC) in mouse cell cultures by ascorbic acid. Nature. 1975;254:531–2.
95. Dahl H, Degre M. The effect of ascorbic acid on production of human interferon and the antiviral activity in vitro. Acta Pathol Scand Sect B. 1976;84:280–4.
96. Mirvish SS, Wallcave L, Eagen M, Shubik P. Ascorbate-nitrate reaction: Possible means of blocking the formation of carcinogenic N-nitroso compounds. Science. 1972;177:65–8.
97. Beetens JR, Hermen AG. Ascorbic acid and Prostaglandin formation. Int J Vitam Nutr Res. 1983;24(Suppl):131s–44s.
98. ElAttar TMA, Lin HS. Effect of vitamin C on prostaglandin synthesis by fibroblasts and squamous carcinoma cells. Prostagl Leukotr Essent Fatty Acids. 1992;47:253–7.
99. Reddy VG, Khanna D, Singh N. Vitamin C augments chemotherapeutic response of cervical carcinoma beta cells by stabilizing p 53. Biochem Biophys Res Comm. 2001;282:409–15.
100. Mirvish S. Experimental evidence for inhibition of N-Nitroso compound formation as a factor in a negative correlation between vitamin C consumption and the incidence of certain cancers. Cancers Res. 1974;54:1948s–51s.

Chapter 3
Potential Therapeutics for Vitamin C and Cancer

Phase 1 Trials, Case Studies, Retrospective Studies, IV Vitamin C, and Quality of Life

Vitamin C Phase 1 Clinical Trials

High-dose vitamin C has proven to be cytotoxic to a wide variety of cancer cell lines [1–5], as well as to boost the cytotoxicity of several common chemotherapy drugs. This has been further confirmed in animal studies, where vitamin C decreased the growth rates of liver, ovarian, pancreatic, and glioblastoma tumors with dosages easily achievable in humans [6–9].

There have been a number of clinical trials done with Intravenous vitamin C in cancer patients. Phase I trials are to be designed to evaluate the safety and tolerability of a new drug, while Phase II trials are designed to evaluate the effectiveness of the treatment.

Riordan et al. conducted a pilot clinical study in 24 late-stage terminal cancer patients [10]. Patients received 0.15–0.71 g intravenous vitamin C per kg body weight per day for up to eight weeks as their sole treatment. Adverse events were minor and the effect on indicators of renal function and blood parameters were minimal; two patients discontinued intravenous vitamin C, one patient had stabilized disease during the trial and continued treatment for 48 weeks. Noteworthy, applied doses of vitamin C were low and plasma concentrations did not exceed 3.8 mM.

Hoffer et al. performed a dose-finding Phase I and pharmacokinetic study in 24 patients with advanced cancer or hematologic malignancy refractory to standard therapy [11]. Patients received 0.4–1.5 g intravenous vitamin C per kg body weight three times weekly for up to 30 weeks as only treatment. High-dose intravenous vitamin C was found to be safe and free of relevant toxicity. Patients receiving 0.6 g or more of vitamin C per kg body weight maintained a good quality of life throughout the trial, while patients receiving the lowest dose experienced deterioration. No patient experienced an objective anticancer response.

© The Author(s) 2014
M.J. Gonzalez and J.R. Miranda-Massari, *New Insights on Vitamin C and Cancer*, SpringerBriefs in Cancer Research, DOI 10.1007/978-1-4939-1890-4_3

Yeom et al. investigated health-related quality of life after intravenous administration of high-dose vitamin C in 39 terminal cancer patients [12]. All patients received 10 g of vitamin C intravenously with a 3-day interval combined with a daily oral intake of 4 g for a week. After administration of vitamin C, patients reported significantly higher scores for physical, emotional, and cognitive function, and significantly lower scores for fatigue, nausea/vomiting, pain, and appetite loss; the other function and symptom scales were not significantly changed.

Monti et al. recruited 14 subjects with metastatic pancreatic cancer to evaluate intravenous vitamin C in combination with standard treatment of gemcitabine (1,000 mg/m2 intravenously, once weekly for 7 weeks) and erlotinib (100 mg orally per day for 8 weeks) in an open-label, dose-escalating Phase I trial [13].

Patients received three infusions per week of intravenous vitamin C (50, 75, or 100 g) for 8 weeks. Nine subjects completed the study (three in each dosage tier): seven subjects had stable disease, while the other two had progressive disease. Pharmacologic vitamin C concentrations were achieved and no increased toxicity was revealed with the addition of ascorbic acid to gemcitabine and erlotinib in pancreatic cancer patients.

Stephenson et al. [14] also conducted a phase 1 study. The primary purpose of this study was to evaluate the safety and tolerability of vitamin C given intravenously.

The second and third purposes of conducting this study were to observe any evidence of tumor response to vitamin C and compare the level of fatigue (weakness), pain control, ability to perform, and quality of life, before and after IV vitamin C was given.

Drisko et al. are conducting a Phase I study in 2 parts to examine safety and pharmacokinetics of escalating doses of intravenous ascorbic acid, first in healthy volunteers followed by evaluation in oncology patients. The study will be conducted at the Infusion Clinic at the University of Kansas Medical Center in conjunction with the Program of Integrative Medicine, Kansas Cancer Research Institute, Department of Pharmacy, Department of Medical Oncology, the Division of Surgical Oncology, and with consultants from the NIH and FDA [15].

Case Series/Studies

Cameron and Campbell [16] reported 50 case reports for advanced cancer patients receiving intravenous and/or oral vitamin C doses (5–45 g per day, indefinitely) as their only treatment. Three patients were reported to experience cytostasis and five had tumor regression, while tumor hemorrhage and necrosis were observed in four cases. Overall, there was an improvement in patients' quality of life and no major side effects were observed. However, some of the patients who experienced a positive effect on tumor growth did receive oral vitamin C instead of intravenous, while the treatment period was short and the dosage was rather low compared to more recent studies.

Riordan et al. published case reports for eight patients with metastasized cancers [17–21]. Vitamin C infusions, as sole treatment or combined with conventional therapy, were generally started at 15 g twice weekly and increased to 30–100 g twice weekly for long periods of time. In all but one case, complete remission was observed. Overall, results indicated lack of toxicity.

Drisko et al. described two cases of advanced epithelial ovarian cancer [22]. Both patients were first treated with chemotherapy and oral antioxidants, after which 60 g intravenous vitamin C was administered twice weekly for one patient in combination with consolidation paclitaxel chemotherapy. Both patients were disease-free three years after diagnosis. No toxicity was found.

Padayatty et al. applied the NCI Best Case Series guidelines to three well-documented cases of advanced cancers, which were confirmed by histopathologic review [23]. Patients received 15–65 g intravenous vitamin C twice weekly for at least two months and lower treatment frequencies thereafter, as their only cancer therapy. In all three cases, remission of cancer was observed.

Noteworthy, for all the successful IV vitamin C case reports, alternative explanations for cancer remission are possible, e.g., remission due to the therapy received before intravenous vitamin C was initiated. Moreover, a general weakness of case reports is that they omit the number of patients having received high-dose intravenous vitamin C without any effect.

Retrospective Studies

Cameron and Pauling performed two controlled retrospective studies comparing 100 terminal cancer patients receiving 10 g vitamin C per day (intravenously for about 10 days and orally thereafter, or only oral) with 1,000 historical control patients that had not received vitamin C. A fourfold-increased average survival time was found in the vitamin C-treated group [24, 25]. In a database analysis comparing 294 incurable cancer patients having received the above-mentioned vitamin C regimen with 1,532 that did not, about twofold longer survival was found in the vitamin C-treated group [26]. The study designs were criticized as they were not randomized nor placebo controlled. Moreover, some patients were treated with oral vitamin C, the treatment period with intravenous vitamin C was only about 10 days, and the doses were rather low.

Vollbracht et al. evaluated the safety and efficacy of intravenous vitamin C administration in the first postoperative year of women with breast cancer, in an epidemiological retrospective cohort study [29].

Data from 125 patients were selected of which 53 were treated with intravenous vitamin C (7.5 g once weekly for a minimum of 4 weeks) additional to standard tumor therapy, and 72 did not receive additional vitamin C. Administration of intravenous vitamin C resulted in a significant reduction of complaints induced by the disease and chemo- or radiotherapy. No side effects resulted by intravenous vitamin C administration, and no effect on tumor status was seen after 6 or 12 months.

In human trials, this therapy has been shown to significantly improve quality of life for breast cancer patients and for patients of multiple other cancers [12–14, 24–26, 29–32].

Another study showed that IV vitamin C significantly reduced inflammation markers in 76 % of cancer patients, which is important for a better prognosis of the disease. Just as impressively, the same trial showed that IV vitamin C decreased tumor markers in 77 % of prostate cancer patients and 73 % of breast cancer patients [34].

Vitamin C and Quality of Life

Vitamin C has been used in cancer patients either as the only therapeutic intervention or in combination with other antineoplastic agents. There are four* published clinical studies were the response and toxicity of vitamin C used alone was tested in cancer patients. In Table 3.1, we summarize 4 case reports of cancer patients where vitamin C was used without any other antineoplastic agents. In Table 3.2, we summarize the information of the clinical studies in cancer patients were vitamin C was used without other antineoplastic agents. The table presents 9 publications, but one of them is a re-evaluation of the data previously published.

Table 3.1 Published case reports using vitamin C without antineoplastic agents

Diagnosis/number of patients	Vitamin C dose	Result	References
Histologically proven reticulum cell sarcoma (1 pt)	Large doses of ascorbic acid	Very dramatic regression of all parameters of disease activity	[35]
		Reduction in dosage coincided with reactivation of the disease	
		Reinstitution of regular high-dose AA induced a second complete remission	
Reticulum cell sarcoma (1 pt)	Mega ascorbic acid therapy	Successfully treated papillary	[36]
		Developed thyroid carcinoma	
42-year-old man with histologically proven widely disseminated reticulum cell sarcoma (1 pt)	Intravenous high-dose ascorbate administration	Two, complete spontaneous regressions	[37]
3 well-documented cases of advanced cancers, confirmed by histopathologic review	High-dose intravenous vitamin C therapy	Patients had unexpectedly long survival times	[26]

Table 3.2 Published clinical studies of vitamin C alone in cancer

Diagnosis/number of patients	Antineoplastic agent	Vitamin C dose	Result	References
Terminal cancer in 100 patients	Not undergoing chemotherapy	10 gm IV qd × 10 days then PO	Four-fold increase in their life expectancy with AA. Better QoL with AA	[24]
Re-evaluation of previous study	Using a different definition of ST	(Survival time)	Increased survival time still found	[25]
150 patients advanced cancer randomized	Not undergoing chemotherapy. Vitamin C or placebo	10 gm po qd (only oral)	No appreciable difference in changes in symptoms, performance status, appetite or weight or survival	[27]
150 patients advanced cancer randomized	Not undergoing chemotherapy. Vitamin C or placebo	10 gm po qd (only oral)	None had objective improvement	[28]
Terminal cancer in 124 patients	Not undergoing chemotherapy	Low AA (0.5–3 gm/d) High AA (5–30 gm/d)	Significantly improved survival (in days). In high AA versus low AA dose. Better QoL in high-AA	[33]
Twenty-four late stage terminal cancer patients	Not undergoing chemotherapy	Continuous infusions of 150–710 mg/kg/day for up to 8 weeks	Vitamin C therapy produced few minor adverse effects. Kidney stone history is a risk factor	[10]
Terminal cancer 39 patients	Not undergoing chemotherapy	10 g AA iv × 2 q 3-day and then 4 g qd × 1 week	Significantly improved health-related quality of life	[12]
Advanced malignancy 24 patients	Not undergoing chemotherapy	0.4, 0.6, 0.9 and 1.5 g ascorbic acid/kg body weight three times weekly	High-dose IV ascorbic acid was well tolerated. Failed to demonstrate anticancer activity in patients with previously treated advanced malignancies	[11]
15 pts with advanced solid tumors refractory to standard therapy	Not undergoing chemotherapy	70, 90, and 110 g/m^2	4-wk phase I study. QoL appeared to improve at weeks 3 and 4	[14]

The case reports had the importance of documenting the positive therapeutic effects of vitamin C in cancer patients like achieving dramatic regression in parameters of disease activity and also achieving remissions and unexpectedly long survival times [35–38].

A study was conducted with a group of terminal cancer patients receiving vitamin C and their results were compared to the results of another group of patients without vitamin C using a retrospective analysis. The results indicated that the mean survival time was much greater for the ascorbate subjects than for the controls and that it is a safe form of treatment is of definite value in the treatment of patients with advanced cancer. Detractors of this publication claim that since the control group was selected retrospectively, selection bias could have affected the results [24].

In order to respond to this argument, the authors re-evaluated survival times using a different definition. The new analysis was published and the increased survival of the ascorbate-treated patients persisted [25].

At that time, a group from Mayo Clinic conducted two randomized trials [23, 24] to challenge the results of Cameron and Pauling. In both studies, they found no appreciable difference in changes in symptoms, performance status, appetite, weight, or survival curves. They concluded on the basis of both studies, that high-dose vitamin C therapy was not effective against advanced malignant disease. However, the design of both of their studies neglected to use the vitamin C in the intravenous form as in the early studies by Cameron and also by Murata [33] as well as later studies showing valuable results in quality of life [12, 29].

The early patients in the Japanese study by Murata et al. received oral vitamin and gradually increased the dose. As experience and knowledge accumulated, they used the higher doses and the intravenous route of administration. The analysis of their results revealed that vitamin C in high doses produced a significantly higher survival and improved quality of life.

Later on, Yeom [12] and colleagues studied 39 terminal cancer patients to determine the effect of high-dose vitamin C on the quality of life. Patients received two intravenous vitamin C infusions of 10 g with a 3-day interval and then an oral dose 4 g vitamin C daily for a week. Demographic data and changes in patients' quality of life were assessed. Validated questionnaires from the European Organization for Research and Treatment of Cancer and the global health/quality of life scale, health score improved significantly after administration of vitamin C ($p = 0.001$). Despite being such a short study, it is encouraging to see a significant improvement in quality of life in terminal condition.

More recently, Stephenson evaluated much higher doses for safety, pharmacokinetics and tolerability of vitamin C as monotherapy in patients with advanced cancer (solid malignant tumors) [14]. Doses of 70, 90, and 110 g/m^2 maintained levels at or above 10–20 mM for 5–6 h. All doses were well tolerated. No patient demonstrated an objective antitumor response in this 4-week study.

An important finding consistently reported in the vitamin C and cancer studies in humans is the improvement in quality of life which is also an important goal of cancer treatment, and clinical experience shows IV vitamin C consistently achieves this improvement.

A prospective study from Korea [12] that we mentioned earlier showed that this therapy significantly improved quality of life for terminal cancer patients, bringing the global health/quality of life score from 36 to 55 and yielding improvements in physical, emotional, and cognitive functions. Disease symptom severity also decreased across the board, with patients showing significantly less fatigue, nausea/vomiting, pain, and appetite loss.

These results were also achieved in a study in Germany [29], which compared breast cancer patients receiving IV vitamin C and standard therapy together, versus standard therapy alone. Those receiving IV vitamin C experienced a marked reduction (nearly 50 %) in unpleasant symptoms and chemo/radiotherapy side effects such as loss of appetite, fatigue, depression, sleep disorders, dizziness, and hemorrhagic diathesis. Another three studies, one Mexican [30] and two Italian [31, 32], also reported improved quality of life in cancer patients supplemented with antioxidants which included vitamin C. Before these studies, a Japanese study utilizing IV vitamin C reported longer survival and improved quality of life in terminal cancer patients [33].

In the USA, a survey showed that over 8,800 patients were treated with IV vitamin C in 2,008, using a total of 355,000 dosage vials. But that was just for the healthcare practitioners taking part in the survey. For the same year, manufacturers reported sales of 855,000 vials of vitamin C. This implies that as many as 21,000 patients received IV vitamin C therapy in 2008 [39].

Several ongoing clinical trials using IV vitamin C to treat cancer will be completed between 2013 and 2014, while some others are recruiting [40]. Therefore, further significant knowledge on various specific aspects of the use of vitamin C in cancer is expected to be generated and published during the next few years. But until then, clinical evidence already shows that this therapy can, at the very least, significantly improve cancer patients' quality of life. Oncologists should therefore strongly consider incorporating this therapy to the standard clinical practice.

Vitamin C, Chemotherapy, and Radiotherapy

If a patient with cancer is about to receive chemo- or radiation therapy, the question of whether the use of vitamin C will be helpful or harmful is important. The only responsible way to answer this question is to carefully and rationally examine all the available evidence. When examining the published evidence on the use of vitamin C in cancer chemo- and radiotherapy, there are many issues that need to be addressed. Does vitamin C interferes with the efficacy of cancer chemo/radiotherapy? Does the blood concentration of vitamin C make a difference in patients with cancer? Is there is a way to give both (vitamin C and chemo) to maximize efficacy (augmenting cancer cell killing of standard anti-neoplastic agents) and minimize toxicity of the treatment to the patient? These are some of the questions that we should address. Since vitamin C is not produced in the body, it must be consumed to avoid low levels associated with sub-optimal physiological functioning and increased risk of disease or mortality.

The high incidence of gastrointestinal problems caused by chemotherapy leading to malnutrition and the cachexia caused by malignancy, depression, and mucosal atrophy of the small intestine leading to malabsorption are important risk factors leading to low vitamin C levels in the patient with cancer and even scurvy. A report of 6 patients with cancer demonstrated that all of them had a low serum vitamin C concentration, and their clinical disorder improved with daily administration of 2 grams of vitamin C.

In patients with malignancy, bleeding and gingivitis are not necessarily caused by the disease or treatment but could be secondary to scurvy. Worsening and death may occur if this diagnosis is missed and failed to be treated [41].

Low vitamin C levels even scurvy should be considered in patients with cancer. A study conducted in 50 patients with advanced cancer measured ascorbic acid concentration in blood and found that 30 % were deficient (<11 μM) and 42 % had low (11.1–23 μM) concentrations. Low plasma vitamin C concentrations were associated with shorter survival [41].

The Antioxidant and Chemotherapy Debate in Cancer Treatment: The Modern Controversy

Vitamin C in cancer therapy stirs controversy. But the focus is not only on whether vitamin C brings a survival edge, but whether it enhances or undermines standard cancer therapies. There has been a concern that antioxidants might reduce the effectiveness of chemotherapy and radiation by reducing the potency of free radicals necessary for cell killing. This misconception is important because it may prevent clinicians from utilizing ascorbate as adjuvant therapy for cancer. In relation to vitamin C, this misconception was due in part to a paper published by Agus, Vera, and Golde in 1999 [42], in which they described how cancer cells acquire and concentrate vitamin C.

The authors suggest that this increased intracellular concentration of ascorbate may provide malignant cells with a metabolic advantage. This suggestion has been embraced by most practitioners without question, resistance, or further evaluation. There are important details that need to be discussed in order to better understand and bring light to this modern controversy.

In general, in one camp are physicians who believe that vitamin C could derail the beneficial effects of chemotherapy or radiation. In another camp are scientists who argue that high doses of antioxidants including vitamin C, may not only protect normal cells during cancer treatment, but may actually help fight tumors. Complicating this situation is the lack of controlled clinical trials, coupled with the unknown applicability of the laboratory findings to actual human cancer patients.

A Memorial Sloan-Kettering news release in 1999 stated that it is possible that taking large amounts of vitamin C could interfere with the effects of chemotherapy or radiation therapy. This statement was in reference to the paper that Dr. David Golde, along with David Agus, MD, and Juan C. Vera, PhD, all of Memorial Sloan-Kettering, had published in Cancer Research [42]. In this paper, it was shown that the vitamin C structure is similar to glucose and that it uses the same transporters to get into the cell. Tumor cells have an increased number of glucose transporters, which is a known characteristic of cancer. Cancer cells use glucose as its main energy fuel. To provide enough glucose, the cancer cell has increased a number of facilitative glucose transporters (GLUTs). Since vitamin C and glucose have similar molecular structure, cellular intake of vitamin C is favored in malignant cells. Certain specialized cells can transport ascorbic acid directly through a sodium ascorbate co-transporter, but in most cells, vitamin C enters through GLUTs in the form of dehydroascorbic acid, which is then reduced intracellularly and retained as ascorbic acid [42]. Ascorbic acid not only acts as an antioxidant, but also has cytotoxic effects at higher concentrations in cancer cells since ascorbic acid at high concentrations has pro-oxidant effects (please refer to the section on Primary Anticancer Mechanisms of Vitamin C in this book).

In their conclusion, Golde et al. stated that an increased intracellular concentration of vitamin C may have effects on tumor growth and in the tumor's ability to respond to oxidative stress associated with chemotherapy and radiation.

In addition to stimulation of the immune system and other metabolic functions, vitamin C in nutritional doses acts mainly as an antioxidant to protect tissues from cellular damage caused by free radicals. Oxidative mechanisms, however, are one way in which chemotherapy and radiation therapy inhibit the growth of cancerous cells. Hence, the reasoning, if many standard cancer treatments act by promoting oxidation, then increasing an antioxidant such as vitamin C during standard cancer treatment will be therapeutically counterproductive and of benefit to the tumor.

In multiple laboratory experiments since 1980, Prasad et al. at the University of Colorado found that high doses of antioxidants such as vitamin C not only can protect normal cells during cancer treatment but also can help fight tumors [43]. In this way, antioxidants may actually improve standard cancer therapy. Prasad explains that the vitamins are selective, inhibiting only the growth of cancer cells.

The hypothesis here is that those normal cells have a homeostatic control for the uptake of antioxidants such as vitamins C and E. So you can provide high doses of these antioxidants and normal cells acquire only what's necessary for their function.

The cancer cells, however, seem to lack this mechanism of control of antioxidant uptake, and therefore, antioxidants accumulate at a higher level. When it accumulates in cancer cells, the intracellular excess initiates a series of epigenetic events which results in cell death (apoptosis), growth inhibition, or re-differentiation.

It is not surprising that scientists would see destruction of cancer cells following administration of vitamin C in vitro. This process is known as the Fenton reaction, in which metal ions, when combined with a reducing agent such as ascorbate, lead to a cycle that causes cellular damage. Some scientists are not sure that the Fenton reaction can occur in the body because there is relatively no free metal ions; copper and iron tend to be bound in vivo. Nevertheless, the Fenton reaction seems to occur in the body, since there are free metal ions in plasma, in the brain, in all organs especially in the disease state. And if vitamin C is present, it will interact with iron, copper, or manganese. It is an experimental and clinical fact, that antioxidants at high doses are selective for inhibiting the growth of cancer cells [43, 44]. Moreover, we must remember that vitamin C in large doses may show a pro-oxidant activity.

Another truth is that large, well-designed clinical trials on the use of antioxidants during chemotherapy and radiation are lacking. Nevertheless, we should mention that of more than 2,300 studies and nearly 5,000 patients reviewed, not a single study showed any clinical evidence of antioxidant use interfering with chemo- therapy [44]. Moreover, the preponderance of the evidence points to a synergistic therapeutic effect in most cases. When antioxidants are included in a person's therapeutic regimen, toxicity is reduced and the patient is more successful at adhering to their chemotherapy regimen [44]. As Dr. Keith Block states, we should ask "What makes better biological sense and what will provide better clinical results?" [44].

In vitro studies have shown that vitamin C in high concentrations (but not low concentrations) enhances the cytotoxicity of 5-FU in a dose-dependent manner in mouse lymphoma [45]. Data show that dietary antioxidants administered in high doses inhibit the growth of cancer cells but not normal cells may improve the efficacy of radiation therapy [46]. Antioxidant vitamins individually or in combi- nation enhance the growth-inhibitory effects of x-irradiation, chemotherapeutic agents on tumor cells in vitro. These cofactors, independently reduce the toxicity of several standard antineoplastic agents on normal cells [46].

A case report on two patients with ovarian cancer stage IIIC documented good response to treatment of chemotherapy along with high-dose antioxidants. Both patients received intravenous vitamin C at a dose sufficient to maintain a plasma concentration above 200 mg/dL. Both had normalization of their CA-125 during the first cycle of chemotherapy, and after 3 years after diagnosis, there was no evidence of recurrence of the disease. One of the patients declined further chemotherapy after the first round and continued on intravenous vitamin C and oral supplementation of several antioxidants and a multivitamin/mineral [47].

A vast body of literature exists on this topic and is summarized in a series of articles by Lamson and Brignall [48–50]. These articles indicate that antioxidants including ascorbate provide beneficial effects in various types of cancers without reduction of efficacy of chemotherapy nor radiation. In addition, the data show increased effectiveness of conventional cancer therapeutic agents when given with antioxidants as well as a decrease in adverse effects [47–51]. Moreover, an article by Prasad et al. [52] shows similar positive results for the combination of antiox- idants and conventional treatment. For a more complete review of the topic, see Moss, 2000 [53].

It has been demonstrated that chemotherapy as well as radiotherapy induce a fall in plasma antioxidants in cancer patients [54–56]. Extensive in vitro studies and limited in vivo studies have revealed that individual antioxidants induce cell dif- ferentiation and growth inhibition to various degrees in rodent and human cancer cells [52]. In addition, Prasad et al. [57] have shown that high-dose multiple antioxidants work synergistically in reducing tumor growth of human parotid acinar cells in vitro [57]. Finally, a clinical trial in Japan with 99 patients showed that terminal cancer patients receiving large doses of AA had much longer survival time (43 versus 246 days) than patients using low ascorbic acid doses [58].

When patients are told that they have cancer, most of them will choose a medical oncologist to guide and manage their condition because they have specialty training in the management of cancer. The recommendations given by the oncologist are based on the results of clinical trials, where patients have received chemotherapy, radiation, and surgery. Since the treatment guidelines have been developed using trials where vitamin C was not included, the use of vitamin C is not recommended because for most practitioners it would become an unknown variable. However, when looking at the outcomes of over 55 years of research in cancer and over 200 billion dollars [59], it is very disappointing to realize that in the last 50 years, while there has been a decrease in mortality from heart disease of 64 % and decrease mortality of cerebrovascular diseases of 74 %, also a decrease in deaths by influenza and pneumonia of 58 % and for cancer of only 5 % [60]. It would seem obvious that we need to do something different to improve outcomes.

Cancer patients with unfavorable prognosis that are having limited or poor response or not tolerating standard therapy may benefit from using concomitant vitamin C therapy.

Current medical practices should be based in the best available evidence. Here, we review the available in vitro, in vivo, and clinical studies of vitamin C during oncological chemotherapy and radiotherapy.

In Vitro/In Vivo Studies

Many in vitro studies have demonstrated synergism between ascorbate and several antineoplastic agents. (See Table 3.3) In some cases, the effect is not related to direct killing effect of ascorbate on the cancer cell, but to increase in the sensitivity of the cell to the antineoplastic agent even in cases of chemotherapy-resistant cells. There are several mechanisms that have been proposed and researched to explain the synergistic effect between antineoplastic agents and vitamin C. These include:

1. Restoration of reduced drug uptake in resistant cells,
2. Modulation of transcription factor AP-1,
3. Stabilization P53,
4. Decrease telomerase activity,
5. Cell-cycle arrest,
6. Cell death/apoptosis,
7. Inhibition of translocation of NF-kappaB and AP-1,
8. Production of H_2O_2, oxidative stress and necrotic cell death.

Beside the independent cytotoxic activity that vitamin C can exhibit in certain conditions, the capacity to sensitize cancer cell to antineoplastic agents to which there was previous resistance has been documented.

The use of ascorbate increases the sensitivity of neuroblastoma cells to 5-FU, Bleomycin x-irradiation but not to methotrexate and DTIC [61]. Ascorbate was also found increased cytotoxic effect of doxorubicin to human breast carcinoma [62].

Doxorubicin (DOX), cisplatin (DDP), and paclitaxel (Tx) were tested alone or in combination for cytotoxicity in two human breast carcinoma cell lines (MCF-7 and MDA-MB-231) [63]. Both cell lines were resistant to DOX. Both cell lines were sensitive to Tx. When ascorbate was tested in combination with the antineoplastic at two concentrations, non cytotoxic (1 microMol) and cytotoxic (100 microMol), both concentrations were found to improve the cytotoxicity of all antineoplastic agents significantly [63]. The in vitro study demonstrated that the concentration required to achieve a cytotoxic effect varies according to the cell line, to the antineoplastic agent in use and to the concentration of ascorbate.

Vitamin C has demonstrated the ability to enhance the chemo-responsiveness of certain cancer cells to 5FU [46]. Vitamin C was tested in vitro on mouse lymphoma, chemo-resistant HEp-2 and human lung fibroblast cell lines [46]. Vitamin C increased the cytotoxicity of 5FU against fibroblast dose-dependently [46]. For the chemo-resistant HEp-2 cell line, only the highest concentration of AA increased the cytotoxicity of 5 FU [46]. It was demonstrated that the combination of ascorbate and 5FU increased the apoptotic effect on the mouse lymphoma. This effect also occurred with the HEp-2 but was less marked and only at a high concentration. These findings suggest that vitamin C at high doses has a chemo-sensitizing effect on certain cancer cell lines that seems to be related to increase in the apoptotic mechanisms.

Since human papilloma virus is frequently associated with cervical cancer, the ability of vitamin C reducing the viral transcription and the effect on cervical carcinoma cell was investigated [64]. It was found that vitamin C down-regulates the redox sensitive transcription factor AP-1 and reduction in one of its transcription targets, and stabilizes P53. It was found that vitamin C increases sensitivity to cisplatin, and etoposide on cervical carcinoma cells by stabilizing P53 using vitamin C is a novel approach and has potential clinical relevance [64].

The cytotoxic effect of the combination of vitamin C on cisplatin and 5-FU was measured on esophageal cancer cell lines OE33 and SKGT-4 [65]. When vitamin C was used along 5-FU or cisplatin, it exerted a significantly enhanced cytotoxic effect compared to either drug individually. This effect was associated in part to inhibition of translocation of NF-kappaB and AP-1, and sensitization of cancer cells to drug-induced cell death [65]. Therefore, vitamin C use may enhance the efficacy of chemotherapy cisplatin and 5-FU when used for the treatment of esophageal cancer [65].

Pharmacologic or nutritional concentrations of ascorbate do not inhibit the activity of antineoplastic agents. In fact, the preponderance of the evidence demonstrates additive or synergistic effects [66]. Verrax et al. assessed the interference of ascorbate with an agent representing each of the five major classes of antineoplastic agents [66].

1. Etoposide (non-intercalating topoisomerase targeting drug).
2. Cisplatin (alkylating agent).

3. 5-Fluorouracil (antimetabolite).
4. Doxorubicin (intercalating topoisomerase targeting drug).
5. Paclitaxel (microtubule-targeting drug).

The experiment was conducted on various cancer cell lines (MCF-7, DU-145, and T24) using ascorbate alone and each drug at half maximal effective concentration (EC50) without ascorbate and in combination with ascorbate at either physiologic (50 μM) concentration or pharmacological concentrations (4.5 mM). The cancer cell lines were exposed for 2 h to the ascorbate and drugs, a protocol that mimics parenteral use [66].

1. Ascorbate alone
2. Drug (EC50) alone
3. Drug (EC50) + ascorbate 50 μM
4. Drug (EC50) + ascorbate 4.5 mM

It was found that the combination of physiologic ascorbate and drug had a small improvement in the (cytolytic) effect of the drug, but pharmacologic ascorbate along with the drug was significantly more effective than the drug alone [66]. Therefore, the results from these experiments suggest that pharmacologic ascorbate may be useful in the clinical arena to improve the antineoplastic effect of a diverse group of chemotherapeutic agents used in oncology protocols.

Gemcitabine in combination with pharmacologic concentrations of ascorbate resulted in a synergistic cytotoxic response in eight pancreatic tumor cell lines including gemcitabine-resistant cell lines [67]. Pharmacologic ascorbate induces the production of H_2O_2 which may produce synergism which can sensitize cancer cells, overcoming the resistance to gemcitabine monotherapy. In addition to the in vitro cell lines results, when treating mice bearing pancreatic tumor with gemcitabine–ascorbate combinations, it consistently enhanced inhibition of growth compared to gemcitabine alone [67]. A 50 % growth inhibition was achieved in a tumor type not responsive to gemcitabine [67]. These results support the study of pharmacologic ascorbate in adjunctive treatments for cancers prone to high failure rates with conventional therapeutic regimens, such as pancreatic cancer.

Upon testing the cytotoxicity of ascorbate to malignant mesothelioma (MMe) cells in combination with drugs used in MMe therapy, synergistic interactions for ascorbate/gemcitabine and ascorbate/EGCG emerged [68]. Examination of these synergistic interactions using the caspase 3 and lactic dehydrogenase assays revealed increased apoptosis and necrosis rates [68].

In Table 3.3, we summarize the findings of the in vitro studies of the effect vitamin C with various antineoplastic agents; these in some cases include data that help understand the mechanism of the effect. In Table 3.4, we summarize the findings on the animal studies (Table 3.5). Finally, Table 3.6 summarizes the clinical trials of vitamin C in combination with other agents.

Table 3.3 Studies on in vitro interaction of vitamin C and antineoplastic agents

Antineoplastic agent	Cytotoxicity: Increased (I) / Neutral (N) / Decrease (D)	Cell type	Mechanism/comment	Ref. author, year
5-FU, bleomycin x-irradiation	I	Mouse neuroblastoma/glioma cells	Neuroblastoma cells were more sensitive to AA alone or in combination	Prasad 1979; [62]
Methotrexate and DTIC	D			
Vincristine	I	Human non-small cell lung cancer	Restoration of drug uptake in resistant cells	Chiang 1994; [63]
Doxorubicin, cisplatin, and paclitaxel	I	Human breast carcinoma	The increased cytotoxic effect was greater with doxorubicin	Kurbacher 1996; [64]
Cisplatin Etoposide	I	Cervical carcinoma HeLa	Modulation of transcription factor AP-1, stabilization P53, decrease telomerase activity, cell-cycle arrest, cell death/apoptosis	Reddy 2001; [65]
5-FU	I	Mouse lymphoma, HEp-2 and human lung fibroblast cell lines	Increased apoptotic effect	Nagy 2003; [47]
Cisplatin 5-Fu	I	Esophageal cancer cell lines OE33 and SKGT-4	Inhibition of translocation of NF-kappaB and AP-1 and sensitizes cancer cells to drug-induced cell death	Abdel-Latif 2005; [66]
Bortezomib	D	Human lung cancer cells	Vitamin C directly binds to and inactivates bortezomib, independent of its antioxidant activity	Zou 2006; [71]
Etoposide Cisplatin, 5-FU Doxorubicin Paclitaxel	I	Human cancer MCF7 (breast), DU145 (prostate) T24 (bladder)	Production of H_2O_2, oxidative stress and cell death/ reinforced the activity in all 5 drugs	Verrax 2009; [67]
Gemcitabine	I	Eight pancreatic tumor cell lines	75 % of cytotoxicity was mediated by H_2O_2/synergism observed even in gemcitabine-resistant lines	Espey 2011; [68]

(continued)

Table 3.3 (continued)

Antineoplastic agent	Cytotoxicity: Increased (I) Neutral (N) Decrease (D)	Cell type	Mechanism/comment	Ref. author, year
Docetaxel, epirubicin, irinotecan and 5-FU, oxaliplatin and vinorelbine	I	Prostate carcinoma cells	Increased cellular sensitivity toward docetaxel, epirubicin, irinotecan, and 5-FU	Frömberg 2011; [72]
Gemcitabine	I	Malignant mesothelioma (Mme)	Increased apoptosis and necrosis rates	Martinotti 2011; [70]
Cisplatin	I	HCT116 human colon cancer cell line	Enhanced sensitivity and apoptosis via up-regulation of p53	An 2011; [73]
Radiation	I	Glioblastoma multiforme (GBM)	5 mM AA radiosensitize GBM causing more double-strand DNA breaks	Herst 2012; [74]
Gemcitabine	I	Malignant pleural mesothelioma (MPM)	Shift from cell proliferation to apoptosis/synergism	Volta 2013; [75]

Table 3.4 Animal studies on the interaction between vitamin C and antineoplastic agents

Anti-neoplastic	Response (±)	Cell type/model	Comment	Author/year
Whole-body radiation	Selective protection to normal tissues. Increased tolerance to radiation adverse effects (+)	Murine fibrosarcoma	Significantly increased the dose of radiation required to cause adv effects	Okunieff 1991; [76]
Cisplatin	Ascorbic acid enhances the antitumor effect of the drug in dramatic increase the survival time and tumor-free survivors. (+)	Dalton's lymphoma C3H/He mice.	Possible cause of the improvement cytotoxic effect may be improved permeability of tumor cell membrane allowing more drug uptake into tumor cells	Sarna 1993; [77]
Bortezomib	Decreased MM cell cytotoxicity (−)	Anti-multiple mye-loma mice	Oral administration	Perrone 2009; [78]
Cyclophos-phamide	Further changes in tumor cells showing dis-integration in the cell membrane, disruption in the nuclear membrane and disruption in the mitochondrial cristae. (+)	Dalton's lymphoma tumor cells /Mice	Decrease in reduced glutathione (GSH)	Prassad 2010; [79]
Gemcitabine	Enhanced growth inhibition up to 50 % in a tumor type not responsive to gemcitabine. (+)	PAN-02 or PANC-1 pancreatic cancer cells. Tumor xeno-grafts athymic mice	Combinations with AA were superior in reducing tumor than gemcitabine alone	Espey 2011;80
Paclitaxel	Increased antitumor effect/1.7-fold higher anticancer effect. 1.6-fold higher viability of normal cells. (+)	H1299 NSC lung cancer cell line/BALB/c mice	Implanted with/without sarcoma. *Mice did not exhibit the typical side effects seen with paclitaxel alone	Park 2012; [81]
Gemcitabine	Strongly reduced the size of primary tumor as well as the number and size of metastases, and prevented hemorrhage. (+)	Malignant pleural mesothelioma (MPM)/Mice	Combination blocked tumor progression and metastasization	Volta 2013; [75]

Table 3.5 Published case reports using antineoplastic agents with vitamin C

Diagnosis/number of patients	Antineoplastic agent	Vitamin C dose	Result	References
Desmoid tumor (3 pts)	Indomethacin	Large doses of ascorbic acid	Improved response in 2 cases	[82]
Stage IIIC advanced ovarian malignancies (2 pts)	Carboplatinum/ paclitaxel	3,000–9,000 mg po daily	Well tolerated	[22]
			Normalization of her CA-125	
			Good response of combination	
Metastatic cancers (5 pts) and lymphomas (2 pts)	Most received standard chemotherapy	15–100 gm iv 2/wk	Maintained or improved efficacy	[85]
			Reduced toxicity	
Metastatic breast (1), metastatic unknown primary (1), local breast cancer (2), cervix (1)	Chemo- or radiotherapy	Oral AsAG (200 mg/kg) and TMG (1.0 mg/kg)	Prevented side effects, such as, severe nausea, or frequent diarrhea in cancer therapies	[84]
Desmoid tumor invading the brachial plexus	Radiotherapy (60 Gy) and etodolac	With ascorbic acid	Major regression of the mass	[83]

A new malignant human T-cell line-labeled PFI-285 has been isolated from a boy with malignant lymphoma. Morphologically, the cells had characteristics of malignant lymphoid cells. A most unusual characteristic was the pronounced sensitivity of the cells to ascorbic acid. Concentrations down to 50 umol/L killed the cells within hours [69].

Summary of antineoplastic and vitamin C in vitro studies:

1. **Cell types**. In vitro testing included a variety of human and mouse cell lines of including neuroblastoma, non-small cell cancer, cervical carcinoma, lymphoma, esophageal, breast, pancreatic, prostate, colon, and pleural.
2. **Antineoplastic evaluated**. Included radiation, 5-FU, bleomycin, methotrexate dacarbazine vincristine doxorubicin, paclitaxel, cisplatin, etoposide, gemcitabine, taxel, epirubicin, irinotecan, oxaliplatin, and vinorelbine.
3. **Cytotoxicity to tumor cell**. Out of a total of 14 studies, 12 demonstrated that the combination antineoplastic with vitamin C increased cytotoxicity against the tumor cell lines.
4. There were two exceptions to the rule. First, vitamin C in combination with methotrexate or dacarbazine decreased the cytotoxicity in mouse neuroblastoma cells. Second, vitamin C inhibited or abrogated all the tested biological activities of bortezomib.

Table 3.6 Published clinical studies using antineoplastic agents with vitamin C

Diagnosis/number of patients	Antineoplastic agent	Vitamin C dose	Result	References
Head and neck and gastrointestinal cancers (25 patients)	Medroxy-progesterone acetate, celecoxib	Oral nutritional formula with C 500 mg/d	Decrease of ROS and proinflammatory cytokines	[92]
			Improvement of quality of life	
Multiple myeloma (MM) who failed more than 2 different prior regimens (65 pts)	Melphalan, arsenic trioxide	1 g iv days 1–4 then twice/wk	Objective responses in 31 of 65 (48 %)	[93]
			Viable therapeutic option for pts with relapsed or refractory MM	
Head and neck and gastrointestinal cancers (44 patients)	Medroxy-progesterone acetate, celecoxib	Oral nutritional formula with C 500 mg/d	Decrease of ROS and proinflammatory cytokines	[94]
			Improvement of quality of life	
Multiple Myeloma refractory to 3–9 previous treatments (22 patients)	Arsenic trioxide bortezomib for a maximum of eight cycles	AA 1 g iv on days 1, 4, 8, and 11 of a 21-day cycle	ABC regimen was well tolerated	[95]
			Objective positive response rate of 27 %	
Newly diagnosed multiple myeloma (MM) (31 patients)	Bortezomib, ascorbic acid and melphalan (BAM)	Oral ascorbic acid 1 g days 1, 4, 8 and 11	Responses occurred in 23/31 patients (74 %)	[96]
			5 (16 %) complete response	
			3 (10 %) very good response	
Myelodysplastic syndrome and acute myeloid leukemia (13 pts)	Decitabine and arsenic trioxide (phase I study)	1 g iv following ATO	1 complete remission	[97]
			5 patients with stable disease	
Breast cancer pts in UICC stages IIa to IIIb (53 Patients)	Standard tumor therapy for at least 4 weeks	7.5 g iv/wk × 4 weeks	Significant reduction of complaints induced by the disease and chemo/radiotherapy,	[98]
Cervical cancer (103 patients)	Cisplatin and radiotherapy	Daily oral antioxidant formula with 100 mg of AA	Supplementation reduced oxidative stress and	[99]
			Improved QoL	

(continued)

Table 3.6 (continued)

Diagnosis/number of patients	Antineoplastic agent	Vitamin C dose	Result	References
Multiple myeloma (58 patients)	Melphalan iv and ATO iv for 7 days. Then placebo or bortezomib	AA 1 gm iv qd for 7 days	High-dose melphalan was safe and well tolerated	[92, 100]
			No significant improvement in the bortezomib groups	
Newly diagnosed cancer (60 patients)	34 patients concomitant chemotherapy	≥ 50 gm iv × 2/wk, adjusted to levels of 19.4–22.2 mM	High-dose intravenous vitamin C safely improved quality of life	[101]
Metastatic stage IV pancreatic cancer (14 subjects)	Standard treatment of gemcitabine and erlotinib	50–100 gm iv AA 3/wk for 8 weeks cycle	9 completed the study	[102]
			7/9 subjects had stable disease	
			No increased toxicity	
Relapsed, refractory multiple myeloma (10 patients)	Arsenic trioxide Bortezomib	1 gm on days 1 and 8 of a 21-day cycle	4 patients had clinical benefit	[103]
			1 patient achieved a durable partial response	
			No dose limiting toxicities	
Biopsy-proven stage IV pancreatic adenocarcinoma. (9 patients)	Gemcitabine	15–125 g iv 2/wk to achieve postinfusion plasma levels of ≥ 20 mM	Adverse effects were rare	[104]
			Diarrhea & dry mouth	
			Mean survival was 13 months (expected life expectancy was 3–5 mo)	

5. **Antineoplastic effect and mechanisms**. In general, the combination of vitamin C and antineoplastic agents was either partly additive or additive or synergistic, The mechanisms/effects documented included:

   (a) Restoration of tumor cell drug uptake.
   (b) Modulation of transcription factor AP-1.
   (c) Inhibition of translocation of NF-kappaB
   (d) Stabilization of P53.
   (e) Decrease in telomerase activity
   (f) Cell-cycle arrest
   (g) Increased apoptosis
   (h) Radio-sensitization increasing double-strand DNA breaks

6. **Conclusions of in vitro studies**:

   (a) Ascorbic acid-sensitive drug uptake mechanism which is important in mediating VCR resistance per se in human lung cancer cells [62].
   (b) High dose of vitamin C in combination with 5-FU chemotherapy enhances the chemo-responsiveness of cancer cells and serves as a potential sensitizer, especially in chemo-resistant cell lines. One of the mechanisms by which vitamin C potentiates cytostatics could be apoptosis induction [46].
   (c) Ascorbic acid improved the cytotoxicity of doxorubicin, cisplatin, and paclitaxel against human breast carcinoma. The mechanisms by which vitamin C potentiates the cytostatics studied are yet unclear [64].
   (d) Increasing drug sensitivity of cervical carcinoma cells by stabilizing P53 using vitamin C is a novel approach and has potential clinical relevance [65].
   (e) Vitamin C enhances the antitumor activity of 5-FU and cisplatin. The data suggest that vitamin C supplementation may improve the efficacy of chemotherapy for esophageal cancer [66].
   (f) Ascorbate inhibited or abrogated all the tested biological activities of bortezomib [67].
   (g) Pharmacologic concentrations of ascorbate killed various cancer cell lines very efficiently (EC [50] ranging from 3 to 7 mM [66].
   (h) The data support the testing of pharmacologic ascorbate in adjunctive treatments for cancers prone to high failure rates with conventional therapeutic regimens, such as pancreatic cancer [67].
   (i) Data indicate that ascorbate/gemcitabine and ascorbate/EGCG affect synergistically the viability of MMe cells and suggest their possible use in the clinical treatment of this problematic cancer [68].
   (j) Antitumor effects of ascorbate were documented and based on its extracellular action, in the induction of apoptosis, and anti-proliferative effect by inducing cell-cycle arrest. Ascorbate was enhanced the cytostatic potency of various chemotherapeutics, which implicates possible therapeutic benefit during tumor treatment [72].

(k) Ascorbate enhanced the cisplatin sensitivity in human colon cancer cells and induced apoptosis via up-regulation of p53 [73].

(l) Pharmacological concentrations of ascorbate radiosensitize gioblastoma multiforme primary cells to a much greater extent than astrocytes; this large therapeutic ratio may be of clinical significance in radiation-resistant cancers [74].

Animal Studies on the Interaction of Vitamin C and Antineoplastic Agents

Seven animal studies with antineoplastic were conducted in the rodent model in a small variety of cancer cell lines using radiation and 5 common antineoplastic agents. The results and conclusions are shown below.

Summary of antineoplastic and vitamin C in animal studies:

1. **Cell types/model.** In vivo testing included a variety of human and mouse cell lines of including fibrosarcoma, lymphoma, multiple myeloma, pancreatic, NSC lung cancer, malignant mesothelioma.

2. **Antineoplastic evaluated.** Included radiation, cisplatin, bortezomib, cyclophosphamide, gemcitabine, paclitaxel.

3. **Effect.** The combination of ascorbic acid with the antineoplastic in seven animal studies between 1993 and 2013 was found that 5 out of 7 demonstrated improved antitumor effects, prevented metastasis or increased survival. Only one (bortezomib) had a negative effect decreasing the cytotoxicity to multiple myeloma cells in mice.

4. **Tolerability.** In 3 out of 7 studies, it was demonstrated that vitamin C decrease the adverse effect of the antineoplastic. None of the studies demonstrated increased adverse effects.

5. **Conclusions of animal studies:**

   (a) Selective protection to radiation adverse effects to normal tissues not affecting tumor cell response. This suggest that if high-dose ascorbic acid is given before radiation dose could be increased in cancer patients without increasing acute complications but with an expected increase in tumor-control probability [76].

   (b) Ascorbic acid enhances the antitumor effect of cisplatin in vivo resulting in increased life span of tumor bearing mice and tumor-free survivors [77].

   (c) Vitamin C can significantly reduce the activity of bortezomib treatment in vivo which suggests that patients receiving that treatment should avoid taking vitamin C dietary supplements [78].

   (d) The combination treatment with ascorbic acid plus cyclophosphamide caused further changes in tumor cells showing disintegration in the cell

surface membrane, disruption in the nuclear membrane and roundish mitochondria with reduction and disruption in the mitochondrial cristae [79].

(e) Gemcitabine–ascorbate combinations administered to mice bearing pancreatic tumor xenografts consistently enhanced inhibition of growth
compared to gemcitabine alone, produced 50 % growth inhibition in a
tumor type not responsive to gemcitabine, and demonstrated a gemcitabine
dose-sparing effect. These data support the testing of pharmacologic
ascorbate in adjunctive treatments for cancers prone to high failure rates
with conventional therapeutic regimens, such as pancreatic cancer [80].

(f) Taken together, these results suggest that combinational chemotherapy
with vitamin C and paclitaxel not only does not block the anticancer effects
of paclitaxel but also alleviates the cytotoxicity of paclitaxel in vivo and
in vitro [81].

(g) Since the data showed that the active nutrient/drug combination and
treatment is synergistic in vitro on malignant pleural mesothelioma MPM
cells, and blocks in vivo tumor progression and metastasization in REN-
based xenografts, the combination is proposed as a new treatment for
MPM [74].

Studies in Cancer Patients

Case Studies

Two reports with cases of desmoid tumor demonstrated improved response along
with radiotherapy and the use of an anti-inflammatory agent [82, 83]. There is also a
report of 5 cancer patients (metastatic breast [41], metastatic unknown primary [41],
local breast cancer [42], cervix [41] where the use of oral ascorbic acid glucoside
(AsAG) (200 mg/kg) and a-tocopherol monoglucoside (TMG) (1.0 mg/kg) prevented the severe nausea or frequent diarrhea, adverse effects usually associated
with radiotherapy, paclitaxel, or CDDP [84].

Riordan [85–89] and Drisko [90] and reported good tumor response and reduced
adverse effects (toxicity) of chemotherapy when adding vitamin C orally or
intravenously.

Riordan et al. published case reports for eight patients with metastasized cancers
[85–89]. Vitamin C infusions, as sole treatment or combined with conventional
therapy, were generally started at 15 g twice weekly and increased to 30 to 100 g
twice weekly for long periods of time. In all but one case, complete remission was
observed. Overall, results indicated lack of toxicity.

Drisko et al. described two cases of advanced epithelial ovarian cancer [90].
Both patients were first treated with chemotherapy and oral antioxidants, after
which 60 g intravenous vitamin C was administered twice weekly for one patient in
combination with consolidation paclitaxel chemotherapy. Both patients were disease-free three years after diagnosis. No toxicity was found.

Clinical Studies and Reports of Antineoplastic Agents with Vitamin C

We found 13 published clinical studies or reports using antineoplastic agents and vitamin C from 2004 to 2013. The studies were mostly in patients with advanced disease, recurrent or refractory to previous treatments, except for the Japanese trial by Takahashi who had 60 newly diagnosed patients. The cancers treated included several different types such as breast, multiple myeloma, pancreatic and leukemia. These trials used intravenous vitamin C in a wide range that went from 1 g and up to 125 g given daily, twice a week, weekly or according to the chemotherapy cycle schedule. The results from these trials were generally positive. Intravenous vitamin C was well tolerated in all the doses given [91–104].

Monti et al. recruited 14 subjects with metastatic pancreatic cancer to evaluate intravenous vitamin C in combination with standard treatment of gemcitabine ($1,000$ mg/m^2 intravenously, once weekly for 7 weeks) and erlotinib (100 mg orally per day for 8 weeks) in an open-label, dose-escalating Phase I trial [102]. Patients received three infusions per week of intravenous vitamin C (50, 75, or 100 g) for 8 weeks. Nine subjects completed the study (three in each dosage tier), seven subjects had stable disease, while the other two had progressive disease. Pharmacologic vitamin C concentrations were achieved, and no increased toxicity was revealed with the addition of ascorbic acid to gemcitabine and erlotinib in pancreatic cancer patients.

The therapeutic effects of chemotherapy were maintained or improved. In some of the studies, a response was observed in 27 % of patients that had been refractory to numerous previous treatments [93]. In other studies, the vitamin C contributed to decrease the adverse effects from the complications of the disease or the chemotherapy or radiotherapy and also improved the quality of life of patients [98, 101]. And in one study, group using vitamin C had prolonged their mean survival from an expected 3–5 months to a mean survival of 13 months [104].

Given the good tolerability of intravenous vitamin C at a very wide dosing range, the benefit of maintaining or improving the therapeutic effect while reducing the toxicity of the treatment and improving quality of life, sometimes producing responses in unresponsive tumors and may even have a positive effect on survival, it is imperative that more studies are conducted to help define the best use of vitamin C in the management of cancer. Currently over 15 trials are underway in an effort to better understand the role of vitamin C in cancer management. Some of these questions remaining to be answered are as follows:

1. Which cancers are best treated with vitamin C?
2. When should vitamin C be started?
3. What dose of vitamin C should be used?
4. Which specific antineoplastic and vitamin C combination is best for a particular cancer and stage?

References

1. Chen P, Stone J, Sullivan G, et al. Anti-cancer effect of pharmacologic ascorbate and its interaction with supplementary parenteral glutathione in preclinical cancer models. Free Radic Biol Med. 2011;51:681–7.
2. Chen Q, Espey MG, Krishna MC, et al. Pharmacologic ascorbic acid concentrations selectively kill cancer cells: action as a pro-drug to deliver hydrogen peroxide to tissues. Proc Natl Acad Sci U S A. 2005;102:13604–9.
3. Verrax J, Calderon PB. Pharmacologic concentrations of ascorbate are achieved by parenteral administration and exhibit antitumoral effects. Free Radic Biol Med. 2009;47:32–40.
4. Chen Q, Espey MG, Sun AY, et al. Pharmacologic doses of ascorbate act as a prooxidant and decrease growth of aggressive tumor xenografts in mice. Proc Natl Acad Sci USA. 2008;105:11105–9.
5. Frömberg A, Gutsch D, Schulze D, et al. Ascorbate exerts anti-proliferative effects through cell cycle inhibition and sensitizes tumor cells towards cytostatic drugs. Cancer Chemother Pharmacol. 2011;67(5):1157–66.
6. Espey MG, Chen P, Chalmers B, et al. Pharmacologic ascorbate synergizes with gemcitabine in preclinical models of pancreatic cancer. Free Radic Biol Med. 2011;50(11):1610–9.
7. Ong PS, Chan SY, Ho PC. Differential augmentative effects of buthionine sulfoximine and ascorbic acid in As_2O_3-induced ovarian cancer cell death: oxidative stress-independent and -dependent cytotoxic potentiation. Int J Oncol. 2011;38(6):1731–9.
8. Martinotti S, Ranzato E, Burlando B. In vitro screening of synergistic ascorbate-drug combinations for the treatment of malignant mesothelioma. Toxicol In Vitro. 2011;25 (8):1568–74.
9. Herst PM, Broadley KW, Harper JL, et al. Pharmacological concentrations of ascorbate radiosensitize glioblastoma multiforme primary cells by increasing oxidative DNA damage and inhibiting G2/M arrest. Free Radic Biol Med. 2012;52(8):1486–93.
10. Riordan HD, Casciari JJ, González MJ, Riordan NH, Miranda-Massari JR, Taylor P, Jackson JA. A pilot clinical study of continuous intravenous ascorbate in terminal cancer patients. P R Health Sci J. 2005;24(4):269–76.
11. Hoffer LJ, Levine M, Assouline S, Melnychuk D, Padayatty SJ, Rosadiuk K, Rousseau C, Robitaille L, Miller WH Jr. Phase I clinical trial of i.v. ascorbic acid in advanced malignancy. Ann Oncol. 2008;19(11):1969–74.
12. Yeom CH, Jung GC, Song KJ. Changes of terminal cancer patients' health-related quality of life after high dose vitamin C administration. J Korean Med Sci. 2007;22(1):7–11.
13. Monti DA, Mitchell E, Bazzan AJ, Littman S, Zabrecky G, Yeo CJ, Pillai MV, Newberg AB, Deshmukh S, Levine M. Phase I evaluation of intravenous ascorbic acid in combination with gemcitabine and erlotinib in patients with metastatic pancreatic cancer. PLoS One. 2012;7(1): e29794.
14. Stephenson CM, Levin RD, Spector T, Lis CG. Phase I clinical trial to evaluate the safety, tolerability, and pharmacokinetics of high-dose intravenous ascorbic acid in patients with advanced cancer. Cancer Chemother Pharmacol. 2013;72(1):139–46.
15. http://clinicaltrials.gov/ct2/show/NCT01833351?term=pharmacokinetics+and+vitamin+c +and+drisko&rank=1. Accessed 17 Dec 2013.
16. Cameron E, Campbell A. The orthomolecular treatment of cancer. II. Clinical trial of high-dose ascorbic acid supplements in advanced human cancer. Chem Biol Interact. 1974;9:285–315.
17. Riordan H, Jackson J, Schultz M. Case Study: High Dose intravenous Vitamin C in the Treatment of a Patient with Adrenocarcinoma of the Kidney. J Orthomol Med. 1990;5:5–7.
18. Jackson JA, Riordan HD, Hunninghake RE, Riordan N. High Dose intravenous Vitamin C and Long Time Survival of A Patient with Cancer of Head of the Pancreas. J Orthomol Med. 1995;10:87–8.

19. Riordan N, Jackson J, Riordan HD. Intravenous Vitamin C in A Terminal Cancer Patient. J Orthomol Med. 1996;11:80–2.

20. Riordan HD, Jackson JA, Riordan NH, Schultz M. High-dose intravenous Vitamin C in the Treatment of a Patient with Renal Cell Carcinoma of the Kidney. J Orthomol Med. 1998;13:72–3.

21. Riordan NH, Riordan HD, Casciari JJ. Clinical and Experimental Experiences with Intravenous Vitamin C. J Orthomolec Med. 2000;15(4):201–13.

22. Drisko JA, Chapman J, Hunter VJ. The use of antioxidants with first-line chemotherapy in two cases of ovarian cancer. J Am Coll Nutr. 2003;22(2):118–23.

23. Padayatty SJ, Riordan HD, Hewitt SM, Katz A, Hoffer LJ, Levine M. Intravenously administered vitamin C as cancer therapy: three cases. CMAJ. 2006;174(7):937–42.

24. Cameron E, Pauling L. Supplemental ascorbate in the supportive treatment of cancer: Prolongation of survival times in terminal human cancer. Proc Natl Acad Sci USA. 1976;73(10):3685–9.

25. Cameron E, Pauling L. Supplemental ascorbate in the supportive treatment of cancer: reevaluation of prolongation of survival times in terminal human cancer. Proc Natl Acad Sci U S A. 1978;75(9):4538–42.

26. Cameron E, Campbell A. Innovation vs. quality control: an 'unpublishable' clinical trial of supplemental ascorbate in incurable cancer. Med Hypotheses. 1991;36(3):185–9.

27. Creagan ET, Moertel CG, O'Fallon JR, Schutt AJ, O'Connell MJ, Rubin J, Frytak S. N Engl J Med (1979) Failure of high-dose vitamin C (ascorbic acid) therapy to benefit patients with advanced cancer; A controlled trial. N Eng J Med. 1979;301(13):687–90.

28. Moertel CG, Fleming TR, Creagan ET, Rubin J, O'Connell MJ, Ames MM. High-dose vitamin C versus placebo in the treatment of patients with advanced cancer who have had no prior chemotherapy; A randomized double-blind comparison. N Engl J Med. 1985;312(3):137–41.

29. Vollbracht C, Schneider B, Leendert V, Weiss G, Auerbach L, Beuth J. Intravenous vitamin C administration improves quality of life in breast cancer patients during chemo-/radiotherapy and aftercare: results of a retrospective, multicentre, epidemiological cohort study in Germany. In Vivo. 2011 Nov-Dec;25(6):983–90.

30. Mantovani G, Madeddu C, Macciò A, Gramignano G, Lusso MR, Massa E, Astara G, Serpe R. Cancer-related anorexia/cachexia syndrome and oxidative stress: an innovative approach beyond current treatment. Cancer Epidemiol Biomarkers Prev. 2004;13(10):1651–9.

31. Mantovani G, Macciò A, Madeddu C, Gramignano G, Lusso MR, Serpe R, Massa E, Astara G, Deiana L. A phase II study with antioxidants, both in the diet and supplemented, pharmaconutritional support, progestagen, and anti-cyclooxygenase-2 showing efficacy and safety in patients with cancer-related anorexia/cachexia and oxidative stress. Cancer Epidemiol Biomarkers Prev. 2006;15(5):1030–4.

32. Fuchs-Tarlovsky V, Bejarano-Rosales M, Gutiérrez-Salmeán G, Casillas MA, López-Alvarenga JC, Ceballos-Reyes GM. Effect of antioxidant supplementation over oxidative stress and quality of life in cervical cancer. Nutr Hosp. 2011 Jul-Aug;26(4):819–26.

33. Murata A. Morishige F. Yamaguchi H. Prolongation of survival times of terminal cancer patients by administration of large doses of ascorbate. International Journal for Vitamin and Nutrition Research. 1982;23:101–113.

34. Mikirova N, Casciari J, Riordan N, Hunninghake R. Clinical experience with intravenous administration of ascorbic acid: achievable levels in blood for different states of inflammation and disease in cancer patients. J Transl Med. 2013;11(1):191.

35. Cameron E, Campbell A, Jack T. The orthomolecular treatment of cancer. III. Reticulum cell sarcoma: double complete regression induced by high-dose ascorbic acid therapy. Chem Biol Interact. 1975;11(5):387–93.

36. Campbell A. Development of a papillary thyroid carcinoma in a patient while on high dosage ascorbic acid therapy. Chem Biol Interact. 1980;30(3):305–8.

37. Campbell A, Jack T, Cameron E. Reticulum cell sarcoma: two complete 'spontaneous' regressions, in response to high-dose ascorbic acid therapy. A report on subsequent progress. Oncology. 1991;48(6):495–7.
38. Padayatty SJ, Riordan HD, Hewitt SM, Katz A, Hoffer LJ, Levine M. Intravenously administered vitamin C as cancer therapy: three cases. CMAJ. 2006;174(7):937–42.
39. Padayatty SJ, Sun AY, Chen Q, Espey MG, Drisko J, Levine M. Vitamin C intravenous use by complementary and alternative medicine practitioners and adverse effects. PLoS One. 2010;5:e11414.
40. http://www.clinicaltrials.gov/ct2/results?term=vitamin+c+and+cancer&Search=Search. Accessed on 27 Dec 2013.
41. Fain O, Mathieu E, Thomas M. Scurvy in patients with cancer. BMJ. 1998;316:1661–2.
42. Mayland CR, Bennett MI. Allan K Vitamin C deficiency in cancer patients. Palliat Med. 2005;19(1):17–20.
43. Agus DB, Vera JC, Golde DW. Stand allocation: a mechanism by which tumors obtain vitamin C. Cancer Res. 1999;59:4555–8.
44. Prasad KN, Kumar A, Kochupillai V, Cole WC. High doses of multiple antioxidant vitamins: essential ingredients in improving the efficacy of standard cancer therapy. J Am Coll Nutr. 1999;18:13–25.
45. Hart J. Data support Antioxidant Use during Chemotherapy. Alt Complement Ther. 2012;18:91–7.
46. Prasad KN, Cole WC, Kumar B, Prasad KC. Pros and cons of antioxidant use during radiation therapy. Cancer Treat Rev. 2002;28:79–91.
47. Nagy B, Mucsi I, Molnar J, Varga A, Thurzo L. Chemosensitizing Effect if Vitamin C in Combination with 5-FU. In Vitro. 2003;17:289–92.
48. Drisko JA, Chapman J, Hunter VJ. The use of antioxidants with first line chemotherapy in two cases of ovarian cancer. J Am Coll Nutr. 2003;22:118–23.
49. Lamson DW, Brignall MS. Antioxidants in cancer therapy: their actions and interactions with oncologic therapies. Alt Med Rev. 1999;4:304–29.
50. Lamson DW, Brignall MS. Antioxidants in cancer therapy II: quick reference guide. Alt Med Rev. 2000;5:152–63.
51. Lamson DW, Brignall MS. Antioxidants in cancer III. Alt Med Rev. 2000;5:196–208.
52. Block KI, Koch AC, Mead MN, Tothy PK, Newman RA, Gyllenhaal C. Impact of antioxidant supplementation on chemotherapeutic toxicity: a systematic review of the evidence from randomized controlled trials. Int J Cancer. 2008;123:1227–39.
53. Prasad KN, Kumar A, Kochupillai V, Cole WC. High doses of multiple antioxidant vitamins: essential ingredients in improving the efficacy of standard cancer therapy. J Am Coll Nutr. 1999;18:13–25.
54. Moss RW. Antioxidants against cancer. New York: Equinox Press; 2000.
55. Weijl NI, Hopman GD, Wipkink-Bakker A, Lentjes ES, Beger HM, Clenton FJ, Osanto S. Cisplatin combination chemotherapy induces a fall in plasma antioxidants of cancer patients. Ann Oncol. 1998;9:1331–7.
56. Clemens MR, Muller-Ladner CI, Gey KF. Vitamins during High Dose Chemo and radio therapy. Z Ermahrungwiss. 1992;31:110–20.
57. Schreurs WH, Odink J, Egger RJ, Wedel M, Brunning PF. The influence of radiotherapy and chemotherapy on the vitamin status of cancer patients. In J Vitam Nutr Res. 1985;55:425–32.
58. Prasad KN, Kumar R. Effect of Individual and multiple antioxidant vitamins on growth and morphology of human non-tumorigenic and tumorigenic parotid acinar cell in cultures. Nutr Cancer. 1996;26:11–9.
59. Murata A, Murata A, Morishige F, Yamaguchi H. Polongation of survival times of terminal cancer patients by administration of large doses of Ascorbate. Int J Vitam Nutr Suppl. 1982;23:103–13.
60. Begley S (2008-09-16). Rethinking the war on cancer. Newsweek. Retrieved 2008-09-08.
61. Kolata G (April 23, 2009). Advances elusive in the drive to cure cancer. The New York Times. Retrieved 2009-05-05.

62. Prasad KN, Sinha PK, Ramanujam M, Sakamoto A. Sodium ascorbate potentiates the growth inhibitory effect of certain agents on neuroblastoma cells in culture. Proc Natl Acad Sci USA. 1979;76:829–32.

63. Chiang CD, Song EJ, Yang VC, Chao CCK. Ascorbic acid increases drug accumulation and reverses vincristine resistance of human non-small-cell lung cancer cells. Biochem J. 1994;301:759–64.

64. Kurbacher CM, Wagner U, Kolster B, Andreotti PE, Krebs D, Bruckner HW. Ascorbic acid (vitamin C) improves the antineoplastic activity of doxorubicin, cisplatin, and paclitaxel in human breast carcinoma cells in vitro. Cancer Lett. 1996;103:183–9.

65. Reddy VG, Khanna N, Singh N. Vitamin C Augments Chemotherapeutic Response of Cervical Carcinoma HeLa Cells by Stabilizing P53 Biochem. Biophys Res Commun. 2001;282:409–15.

66. Abdel-Latif MM, Raouf AA, Sabra K, Kelleher D, Reynolds JV. Vitamin C enhances chemosensitization of esophageal cancer cells in vitro. J Chemother. 2005;17(5):539–49.

67. Verrax J, Calderon PB. Pharmacologic concentrations of ascorbate are achieved by parenteral administration and exhibit antitumoral effects. Free Radic Biol Med. 2009;47(1):32–40.

68. Espey MG, Chen P, Chalmers B, Drisko J, Sun AY, Levine M, Chen Q. Pharmacologic ascorbate synergizes with gemcitabine in preclinical models of pancreatic cancer. Free Radic Biol Med. 2011;50(11):1610–9.

69. Helgestad J, Pettersen R, Storm-Mathisen I, Schjerven L, Ulrich K, Smeland EB, Egeland T, Sørskaard D, Brøgger A, Hovig T, Degrt M, Lie SO. Characterization of a new malignant human T-cell line (PFI-285) sensitive to ascorbic acid. Eur J Haematol. 1990 Jan;44(1):9–17.

70. Martinotti S, Ranzato E, Burlando B. Toxicol In Vitro. In vitro screening of synergistic ascorbate-drug combinations for the treatment of malignant mesothelioma. 2011;25 (8):1568–74.

71. Zou W, Yue P, Lin N, He M, Zhou Z, Lonial S, Khuri FR, Wang B, Sun SY. Vitamin C inactivates the proteasome inhibitor PS-341 in human cancer cells. Clin Cancer Res. 2006;12(1):273–80.

72. Frömberg A, Gutsch D, Schulze D, Vollbracht C, Weiss G, Czubayko F, Aigner A. Ascorbate exerts anti-proliferative effects through cell cycle inhibition and sensitizes tumor cells towards cytostatic drugs. Cancer Chemother Pharmacol. 2011;67(5):1157–66.

73. An SH, Kang JH, Kim DH. MS. Vitamin C increases the apoptosis via up-regulation p53 during cisplatin treatment in human colon cancer cells. BMB Rep. 2011;44(3):211–6.

74. Herst PM, Broadley KW, Harper JL, McConnell MJ. Pharmacological concentrations of ascorbate radiosensitize glioblastoma multiforme primary cells by increasing oxidative DNA damage and inhibiting G2/M arrest. Free Radic Biol Med. 2012;52(8):1486–93.

75. Volta V, Ranzato E, Martinotti S, Gallo S, Russo MV, Mutti L, Biffo S, Burlando B. Preclinical demonstration of synergistic Active Nutrients/Drug (AND) combination as a potential treatment for malignant pleural mesothelioma. PLoS One. 2013;8(3):e58051.

76. Okunieff P. Interactions between ascorbic acid and the radiation of bone marrow, skin, and tumor. Am J Clin Nutr. 1991;54:1281S–3S.

77. Sarna S, Bhola RK. Chemo-immunotherapeutical studies on Dalton's lymphoma in mice using cisplatin and ascorbic acid: synergistic antitumor effect in vivo and in vitro. Arch Immunol Ther Exp (Warsz). 1993;41(5–6):327–33.

78. Perrone G, Hideshima T, Ikeda H, Okawa Y, Calabrese E, Gorgun G, Santo L, Cirstea D, Raje N, Chauhan D, Baccarani M, Cavo M, Anderson KC. Ascorbic acid inhibits antitumor activity of bortezomib in vivo. Leukemia. 2009;23(9):1679–86.

79. Prasad SB, Rosangkima G, Nicol BM. Eur J Pharmacol. Cyclophosphamide and ascorbic acid-mediated ultrastructural and biochemical changes in Dalton's lymphoma cells in vivo. 2010;645(1–3):47–54.

80. Espey MG, Chen P, Chalmers B, Drisko J, Sun AY, Levine M, Chen Q. Pharmacologic ascorbate synergizes with gemcitabine in preclinical models of pancreatic cancer. Free Radic Biol Med. 2011;50(11):1610–9.

81. Park JH, Davis KR, Lee G, Jung M, Jung Y, Park J, Yi SY, Lee MA, Lee S, Yeom CH, Kim J. Ascorbic acid alleviates toxicity of paclitaxel without interfering with the anticancer efficacy in mice. Nutr Res. 2012;32(11):873–83.
82. Waddell WR, Gerner RE. Indomethacin and ascorbate inhibit desmoid tumors. J Surg Oncol. 1980;15(1):85–90.
83. Kilçiksiz S, Gökçe T, Somali I, Duransoy A, Aydin A, Yiğit S. Combined administration of ethodolac, ascorbic acid and radiotherapy as adjuvant therapies in an extrathoracic desmoid tumor with gross postoperative residual disease; case report and review of the literature. J BU ON. 2006;11(3):355–338.
84. Koizumi M, Nishimura T, Kagiya T. Clinical trial of adverse effect inhibition with glucosides of vitamin C and vitamin E in radiotherapy and chemotherapy. J Can Res Ther. 2005;1:239.
85. Riordan HD, Riordan NH, Jackson JA, Casciari JJ, Hunninghake R, González MJ, Mora EM, Miranda-Massari JR, Rosario N, Rivera A. Intravenous vitamin C as a chemotherapy agent: a report on clinical cases. P R Health Sci J. 2004;23(2):115–8.
86. Riordan H, Jackson J, Schultz M. Case Study: High Dose intravenous Vitamin C in the Treatment of a Patient with Adrenocarcinoma of the Kidney. J Orthomol Med. 1990;5:5–7.
87. Jackson JA, Riordan HD, Hunninghake RE, Riordan N. High dose intravenous vitamin C and long time survival of a patient with cancer of head of the pancreas. J Orthomol Med. 1995;10:87–8.
88. Riordan N, Jackson J, Riordan HD. Intravenous Vitamin C in A Terminal Cancer Patient. J Orthomol Med. 1996;11:80–2.
89. Riordan HD, Jackson JA, Riordan NH, Schultz M. High-dose intravenous Vitamin C in the Treatment of a Patient with Renal Cell Carcinoma of the Kidney. J Orthomol Med. 1998;13:72–3.
90. Riordan NH, Riordan HD, Casciari JJ. Clinical and Experimental Experiences with Intravenous Vitamin C. J Orthomolec Med. 2000;15(4):201–13.
91. Drisko JA, Chapman J, Hunter VJ. The use of antioxidants with first-line chemotherapy in two cases of ovarian cancer. J Am Coll Nutr. 2003;22(2):118–23.
92. Mantovani G, Madeddu C, Macciò A, Gramignano G, Lusso MR, Massa E, Astara G, Serpe R. Cancer-related anorexia/cachexia syndrome and oxidative stress: an innovative approach beyond current treatment. Cancer Epidemiol Biomarkers Prev. 2004;13(10):1651–9.
93. Berenson JR, Boccia R, Siegel D, Bozdech M, Bessudo A, Stadtmauer E, Talisman Pomeroy J, Steis R, Flam M, Lutzky J, Jilani S, Volk J, Wong SF, Moss R,Patel R, Ferretti D, Russell K, Louie R, Yeh HS, Swift RA. Efficacy and safety of melphalan, arsenic trioxide and ascorbic acid combination therapy in patients with relapsed or refractory multiple myeloma: a prospective, multicentre, phase II, single-arm study. Br J Haematol. 2006;135 (2):174–183.
94. Mantovani G, Macciò A, Madeddu C, Gramignano G, Lusso MR, Serpe R, Massa E, Astara G, Deiana L. A phase II study with antioxidants, both in the diet and supplemented, pharmaconutritional support, progestagen, and anti-cyclooxygenase-2 showing efficacy and safety in patients with cancer-related anorexia/cachexia and oxidative stress. Cancer Epidemiol Biomarkers Prev. 2006;15(5):1030–4.
95. Berenson JR, Matous J, Swift RA, Mapes R, Morrison B, Yeh HS. A phase I/II study of arsenic trioxide/bortezomib/ascorbic acid combination therapy for the treatment of relapsed or refractory multiple myeloma. Clin Cancer Res. 2007 15;13(6):1762–1768.
96. Berenson JR, Yellin O, Woytowitz D, Flam MS, Cartmell A, Patel R, Duvivier H, Nassir Y, Eades B, Abaya CD, Hilger J, Swift RA. Bortezomib, ascorbic acid and melphalan (BAM) therapy for patients with newly diagnosed multiple myeloma: an effective and well-tolerated frontline regimen. Eur J Haematol. 2009;82(6):433–9.
97. Welch JS, Klco JM, Gao F, Procknow E, Uy GL, Stockerl-Goldstein KE, Abboud CN, Westervelt P, DiPersio JF, Hassan A, Cashen AF, Vij R. Combination decitabine, arsenic trioxide, and ascorbic acid for the treatment of myelodysplastic syndrome and acute myeloid leukemia: a phase I study. Am J Hematol. 2011;86(9):796–800.

98. Vollbracht C, Schneider B, Leendert V, Weiss G, Auerbach L, Beuth J. Intravenous vitamin C administration improves quality of life in breast cancer patients during chemo-/ radiotherapy and aftercare: results of a retrospective, multicentre, epidemiological cohort study in Germany. In Vivo. 2011;25(6):983–90.

99. Fuchs-Tarlovsky V, Bejarano-Rosales M, Gutiérrez-Salmeán G, Casillas MA, López-Alvarenga JC, Ceballos-Reyes GM. Effect of antioxidant supplementation over oxidative stress and quality of life in cervical cancer. Nutr Hosp. 2011;26(4):819–26.

100. Sharma M, Khan H, Thall PF, Orlowski RZ, Bassett RL Jr, Shah N, Bashir Q, Parmar S, Wang M, Shah JJ, Hosing CM, Popat UR, Giralt SA, Champlin RE, Qazilbash MH. A randomized phase 2 trial of a preparative regimen of bortezomib, high-dose melphalan, arsenic trioxide, and ascorbic acid. Cancer. 2012;118(9):2507–15.

101. Takahashi H, Mizuno H, Atsuo Yanagisawa A. High-dose intravenous vitamin C improves quality of life in cancer patients. Personalized Med Univ. 2012;1:49–53.

102. Monti DA, Mitchell E, Bazzan AJ, Littman S, Zabrecky G, Yeo CJ, Pillai MV, Newberg AB, Deshmukh S, Levine M. Phase I evaluation of intravenous ascorbic acid in combination with gemcitabine and erlotinib in patients with metastatic pancreatic cancer. PLoS One. 2012;7(1): e29794.

103. Held LA, Rizzieri D, Long GD, Gockerman JP, Diehl LF, de Castro CM, Moore JO, Horwitz ME, Chao NJ, Gasparetto C. A Phase I study of arsenic trioxide (Trisenox), ascorbic acid, and bortezomib (Velcade) combination therapy in patients with relapsed/refractory multiple myeloma. Cancer Invest. 2013;31(3):172–6.

104. Welsh JL, Wagner BA, van't Erve TJ, Zehr PS, Berg DJ, Halfdanarson TR, Yee NS, Bodeker KL, Du J, Roberts LJ 2nd, Drisko J, Levine M, Buettner GR, Cullen JJ. Pharmacological ascorbate with gemcitabine for the control of metastatic and node-positive pancreatic cancer (PACMAN): results from a phase I clinical trial. Cancer Chemother Pharmacol. 2013;71(3):765–75.

Conclusion

There are a wide variety of mechanisms by which ascorbate prevents and inhibits malignant growth. We have described the ones that seem more relevant, scientifically logical and for which there is the most evidence. The pro-oxidative effect, the contribution to the electron flow in the mitochondrial energy, the anti-inflammatory action, the anti-angiogenic effect, the immune supportive function, and several other factors such as reversion of chemotherapy resistance contributing in a complex multifactorial way to overcome malignancy. It is very likely that many of these mechanisms interplay in ascorbate's anticancer action. The preponderance of the evidence supports the notion of increasing ascorbate in patients suffering malignancies, especially provided by intravenous route as a therapeutic strategy. Ascorbate may produce benefits in both prevention and treatment of cancer, by inhibiting malignant cell proliferation and inducing differentiation [1] and re-differentiation [2]. In addition, ascorbate has been of value in the palliation of pain [3, 4] and as an ergogenic agent [5–7], which can substantially improved the quality of life of terminal cancer patients.

The ideal anticancer agent is obviously one that specifically interferes with tumor growth, prolongs survival time, and improves quality of life. There is evidence that ascorbate fits this description. A protocol for the proper administration of intravenous Vitamin C has been published by our group [8]. Based on the evidence reviewed herein, we suggest the use of high dose intravenous ascorbic acid as adjuvant therapy in cancer treatment and the exploration of new cancer therapies based on modulation of the cellular redox state. Cancer has been viewed as a group of diseases having in common uncontrolled rapidly growing cells leading to the formation of tumors and metastasis, mainly from a genetic origin. The current paradigm has supported surgery, chemotherapy and radiation as main treatments for cancer; which over the last 60 years has produced very limited results. Given the information provided herein about the effect of Vitamin C on cancer, we proposed a change in paradigm in relation to cancer treatment in which cancer should be viewed as a metabolic disease.

© The Author(s) 2014

M.J. Gonzalez and J.R. Miranda-Massari, *New Insights on Vitamin C and Cancer,*
SpringerBriefs in Cancer Research, DOI 10.1007/978-1-4939-1890-4

Appendix
Increasing the Effectiveness of Intravenous Vitamin C as an Anticancer Agent

After over 60 years of experience with vitamin C and Cancer, what can we say about vitamin C as an anticancer agent?

First, the extensive experience and published papers demonstrate that the use of high dose (oral and intravenous) vitamin C is *remarkably safe* [9–15].

Second it confirms that it has many therapeutic benefits such as...

1. Improving quality of life [16–18]:

   a. Decreasing adverse effects of standard cancer treatments
   b. Reducing pain
   c. Increasing energy
   d. Increasing appetite

2. May reduce complications of the disease [19–24]:

   a. Resolving ascorbate's insufficiency in the cancer patient
   b. Combating infections (viral, bacterial, fungi)
   c. Decreasing cancer-associated inflammation
   d. Preventing cancer associated sepsis

3. Pharmacological doses have shown cytostatic or cytotoxic action in cancer cells through a variety of mechanisms [25]:

   a. Fuel control of malignant cells by glucose antagonism
   b. Electron donor for the energy RedOx cancer cell mitochondria problem
   c. Hydrogen peroxide formation
   d. Collagen formation
   e. Immune enhancement
   f. Sustain and possibly improve the cytotoxic effect of standard antineoplastic agents (See Section on Chemotherapy)

© The Author(s) 2014

M.J. Gonzalez and J.R. Miranda-Massari, *New Insights on Vitamin C and Cancer*, SpringerBriefs in Cancer Research, DOI 10.1007/978-1-4939-1890-4

Many patients have shown impressive responses in tumor reduction, improvement in pain control, increased energy level and appetite, in general we can state that most patients improve their quality of life but nevertheless the total success of the use of intravenous vitamin C as an anticancer agent has been variable. This may be due to a number of direct interacting variables.

In order to consistently improve cancer patient outcomes, it is important to have a comprehensive health evaluation that allows identifying contributing factors to health deterioration and the barriers to healing. These must be identified and corrected.

These include but are not limited to:

1. Cell energy-related metabolic derangements in cancer patients [26–28].
2. Toxicities (tobacco, alcohol, pesticides, heavy metals, hydrocarbons, food nitrosamines) [29–36].
3. Medications (Opioids impair immune responses, increase angiogenesis, and may even act directly on tumor cells to encourage their growth and spread. There are epidemiologic, animal, and cellular studies that suggest a role of mu opiod receptors (MOR) on cancer growth and metastasis) [37–39].
4. Hormonal imbalances/endocrine disruptors [40, 41].
5. Excessive inflammation [42, 43].
6. Some infectious agents and the imbalance of the body flora [44, 45].
7. Excessive psychological stress [46, 47].
8. Excessive exposure to radiation [48, 49].

(10 % of invasive cancers are related to radiation exposure, including both ionizing radiation and nonionizing radiation).

Physiological/Cellular Variables to Consider That May Be Relevant to the Effectiveness of IV Vitamin C Therapy

1-Level of Tissue Oxygenation

The level of tissue oxygenation may be an important limiting factor in the anticancer activity of high dose intravenous Vitamin C. As we are well aware of one of the most important mechanisms by which Vitamin C exerts its anticancer action is by the production of hydrogen peroxide. For this to occur, the presence of oxygen is a requisite. Limited oxygen availability reduces the chances of the production of hydrogen peroxide from the conversion of ascorbic acid to dehydroascorbic acid. We propose the utilization of hyperbaric oxygen immediately after IV vitamin C therapy to increase its effectiveness as an anticancer agent to increase the formation of hydrogen peroxide, and therefore enhance the anticancer effect.

In relation to ozone, it is known that Vitamin C is antagonistic to ozone, although it has been shown that ozone does not to break down Vitamin C in the body. Persons taking megadoses of vitamin C should take the ozone treatment first, wait 30 minutes, and then take the Vitamin C.

General Aspects of Oxygenation

Oxygen is a necessary component in every chemical reaction important to human physiology. The appearance of oxygen on our globe induced profound changes in the nature of living systems which with enough energy available started to differentiate and build complex structures with complex functions. Oxidation is loss of electrons to more electronegative group whereas oxygenation is carrying of oxygen molecules. Oxidation was added to fermentation and proliferation was subjected to regulation. Fermentation demanded no structure, being the result of the action of a series of single molecules. Oxidation, with its electron flow, demanded structure and sequential electronic mobility to increase energy production.

Oxygen tension in tissues depends on metabolism and vascular supply, and in tumors, there exist many areas of irregular blood flow. This may be caused by the presence of cells in different stages, or also because the blood capillaries may collapse due to external pressure resulting from unbalanced cell proliferation. This may also be the result of structural defects due to deficient collagen (secondary to ascorbate insufficiency) in the vessel walls, decreased diffusion capacity, and alveolar hypoventilation. These conditions may collectively result in a problem known as hypoxia within cancerous growths, which limits the effectiveness of cancer therapy.

Hypoxia is a critical hallmark of cancer and involves enhanced cell survival, angiogenesis, glycolytic metabolism, and metastasis. Hypoxia has also been shown to increase genetic instability, activate invasive growth, and preserve the undifferentiated cell state [50].

1-Increases Oxygen (Ozone and hyperbaric oxygen)

An Italian group postulates that a prolonged cycle of ozonated autohemotherapy may correct tumor hypoxia, lead to less aggressive tumor behavior. Improving oxygen levels would be expected to favor the anticancer effect of vitamin C [51].

Ozone therapy has been reported to produce an increase in red blood cell glycolysis rate. This leads to stimulation of 2,3-diphosphoglycerate which then allows a rise of the oxygen released to the tissues. Ozone facilitates the Krebs's cycle by improving the oxidative carboxylation of pyruvate and promoting the synthesis of ATP. There is also an increase in antioxidant enzymes that act as free radical scavengers (such as glutathione peroxidase, catalase, and superoxide dismutase) [52]. Vasodilation is also induced by ozone which leads to increased oxygen and nutrients and immune factors available to the cell [53]. Ozonized autohemotransfusion may be useful to improve both the poor rheological properties of the blood and the oxygen delivery to tissues [54] and therefore increase oxygen, immune factors, and nutrients that improve healing and tumor response. Animal studies have shown very significant increased survival in advanced head and neck squamous cell carcinomas with the application of ozone. Although the mechanisms for this effect has not been totally elucidated, it is believed that various important immune-modulatory effects in macrophages, polymorphonuclear cells (PMN), NK cells, and cytotoxic T lymphocytes are involved as well as other metabolic modulatory effects are relevant [55].

Therefore, although at the present time there is no evidence that ozone can improve the anticancer activity of vitamin C, given the scope of its biological effects, it might be important to test this combination. Hyperbaric oxygen (HBO) treatment has been used to treat disorders involving hypoxia and ischemia, by enhancing the amount of dissolved oxygen in the plasma and thereby increasing O_2 delivery to the tissue. HBO might have tumor-inhibitory effects by saturating tumors with oxygen, thus reversing the cancer promoting effects of tumor hypoxia. Reduced cell proliferation, together with a significant change in histology, has been shown after HBO treatment [56]. HBO may increase available oxygen for Vitamin C and potentiate the anticancer activity of ascorbate by increasing the formation of hydrogen peroxide.

2-Increased Oxygen Metabolism

Activates of the Krebs cycle, increases oxidative decarboxylation of pyruvate and ATP production.

Capable of oxidizing the lipid layer of malignant cells and destroy them through cell lysis.

Oxygen reacts with the unsaturated fatty acids of the lipid layer in celllular membranes, forming hydro peroxides. Lipid peroxidation products include peroxyl radicals, vital for killer cell action, these products may also include cytotoxic aldehydes [57].

3-Increases Circulation

Permitting more oxygen, Vitamin C and immune factors delivery to tissues.

4-Decreases Bacteria/Viral/Fungi Load

Microbes are important modulators of the immune system and, if not in an adequate balance they can produce excess inflammation. Since inflammation is known to play a major role in the pathogenesis of cancer, microbial balance can influence tumor progression. This can occur by chronic activation of inflammation, alteration of tumor microenvironment, induction of genotoxic responses, and metabolism [58].

Other Oxygen-Related Compounds

Sodium Bicarbonate

May correct acidosis (increased fermentation), a common physiological characteristic of cancer tissue. Na bicarbonate, also has a specific ability (i.e., not possessed by other basic compounds) to destroy fungi colonies [59, 60].

Dichloroacetic Acid

May improve mitochondrial function by facilitating oxidative phosphorylation which is lacking in the cancer cell [60, 61].

2-Excessive Glucose [62, 63]

Excessive blood glucose can compete with Vitamin C for the glut receptor sites. It is a good therapeutic approach to provide the high dose IV Vitamin C in an empty stomach. Nevertheless, we should be aware that sleepiness and hypoglycemia symptoms may arise. Receiving these IVs causes the body to produce insulin because it believes that the blood sugar is spiking. You might experience hypoglycemia-like symptoms. If you measure your blood sugar during the infusion of IV vitamin C, the meter reads an enormously high number because it thinks the vitamin C is sugar. Be sure to keep available some orange juice in case an hypoglycemic episode ensues.

3-Physiological Red-Ox Balance [64]

The balance between oxidation and anti-oxidation is believed to be critical in maintaining healthy biological systems. Reactive oxygen species (ROS) and reactive nitrogen species (RNS) play important roles in regulation of cell survival. In general, moderate levels of ROS/RNS may function as signals to promote cell proliferation and survival, whereas severe increase of ROS/RNS can induce cell death. Under physiologic conditions, the balance between generation and elimination of ROS/RNS maintains the proper function of redox-sensitive signaling proteins. Normally, the redox homeostasis ensures that the cells respond properly to endogenous and exogenous stimuli. However, when the redox homeostasis is disturbed, oxidative stress may lead to aberrant cell death and contribute to disease development. Redox balance plays a critical role in maintaining the biologic processes under normal conditions. Disruption of redox homeostasis will result in a deregulation of apoptosis associated with various diseases, including cancer, degenerative diseases, and aging. In general, ROS at low levels act as signaling molecules that promote cell proliferation and cell survival. In contrast, a severe increase in ROS can induce cell death. There is a continuous demand for exogenous antioxidants in order to prevent oxidative stress, representing a disequilibrium redox state in favor of oxidation. However, high doses of isolated compounds may be toxic, owing to pro-oxidative effects at high concentrations or their potential to react with beneficial concentrations of ROS normally present at physiological conditions that are required for optimal cellular functioning. All said and done, the physiological Red-Ox state may also influence Intravenous Vitamin C effectiveness as an anticancer agent. We do not recommend the concomitant application of agents with antioxidative potential (such as glutathione, B-Complex vitamins) with intravenous Vitamin C as they may interfere with the oxidative activity of Vitamin C and reduce its anticancer potential.

Common side effects of high dose IV Vitamin C therapy following the Riordan Protocol: Dehydration and, less commonly, blood sugar changes.

References

1. Lee JY, Chang MY, Park CH, Kim HY, Kim JH, Son H, Lee YS, Lee SH. Ascorbate induced differentiation of embryonic cortical precursors into neurons and astrocytes. J Neurosci Res. 2003;73:156–65.
2. Kang JH, Shi YM, Zheng RL. Effects of ascorbic acid in human hepatoma cell proliferation and redifferentiation. Acta Pharmacol Sin. 1999;20:1019–24.
3. Ringsdorf WM, Vitamin C. Supplementation and relief from pain. J Alabama Dental Assoc. 1969;68:47–50.
4. Jensen NH. Reduced pain from osteoarthritis in hip joint or knee joint during treatment with calcium ascorbate. Ugeskr Laeger. 2003;165:2563–6.
5. Komarova SV, Ataullakhanov FI, Globus RK. Bioenergetics and mitochondrial transmembrane potential during differentiation of cultured osteoblasts. Am J Physiol Cell Physiol. 2000;279:c1220–9.
6. Luo G, Xie ZZ, Liu FY, Zhang GB. Effect of vitamin C on mitochondrial function and ATP content in hypoxic rats. Zhongguo Yao Li Xue Bao. 1998;19:351–5.
7. Gonzalez MJ, Miranda-Massari JR, Riordan HD. Vitamin C as an Ergogenic Aid. J Orthomolec Med. 2005;20:100–2.
8. Riordan HD, Hunninghake RB, Riordan NR, Jackson JJ, Meng X, Taylor P, Casciari JJ, Gonzalez MJ, Miranda-Massari JR, Mora EM, Rosario N, Rivera A. Intravenous ascorbic acid: protocol for its application and use. PR Health Sci J. 2003;22:287–90.
9. Murata A, Morishige F, Yamaguchi H. Prolongation of survival times of terminal cancer patients by administration of large doses of ascorbate. Int J Vitam Nutr Res Suppl. 1982;23:103–13.

10. Drisko JA, Chapman J, Hunter VJ. The use of antioxidants with first-line chemotherapy in two cases of ovarian cancer. J Am Coll Nutr. 2003;22(2):118–23.

11. Riordan HD, Casciari JJ, González MJ, Riordan NH, Miranda-Massari JR, Taylor P, Jackson JA. A pilot clinical study of continuous intravenous ascorbate in terminal cancer patients. P R Health Sci J. 2005;24(4):269–76.

12. Hoffer LJ, Levine M, Assouline S, Melnychuk D, Padayatty SJ, Rosadiuk K, Rousseau C, Robitaille L, Miller WH Jr. Phase I clinical trial of i.v. ascorbic acid in advanced malignancy. Ann Oncol. 2008 Nov;19(11):196974.

13. Padayatty SJ, Sun AY, Chen Q, Espey MG, Drisko J, Levine M. Vitamin C: intravenous use by complementary and alternative medicine practitioners and adverse effects. PLoS One. 2010 Jul 7;5(7):e11414.

14. Stephenson CM, Levin RD, Spector T, Lis CG. Phase I clinical trial to evaluate the safety, tolerability, and pharmacokinetics of high-dose intravenous ascorbic acid in patients with advanced cancer. Cancer Chemother Pharmacol. 2013;72(1):139–46.

15. Fowler AA, Syed AA, Knowlson S, Sculthorpe R, Farthing D, DeWilde C, Farthing CA, Larus TL, Martin E, Brophy DF. Gupta S; Medical Respiratory Intensive Care Unit Nursing, Fisher BJ, Natarajan R. Phase I safety trial of intravenous ascorbic acid in patients with severe sepsis. J Transl Med. 2014 Jan;31(12):32.

16. Yeom CH, Jung GC, Song KJ. Changes of terminal cancer patients' health-related quality of life after high dose vitamin C administration. J Korean Med Sci. 2007;22(1):7–11.

17. Vollbracht C, Schneider B, Leendert V, Weiss G, Auerbach L, Beuth J. Intravenous vitamin C administration improves quality of life in breast cancer patients during chemo-/radiotherapy and aftercare: results of a retrospective, multicentre, epidemiological cohort study in Germany. In Vivo. 2011 Nov-Dec;25(6):98390.

18. Takahashia H, Mizunob H, Yanagisawa A. High-dose intravenous vitamin C improves quality of life in cancer patients. Pers Med Univ. 2012;1(1):49–53.

19. Head KA. Ascorbic acid in the prevention and treatment of cancer. Altern Med Rev. 1998;3(3):174–86.

20. Mayland CR, Bennett MI, Allan K. Vitamin C deficiency in cancer patients. Palliat Med. 2005;19(1):17–20.

21. Ichim TE, Minev B, Braciak T, Luna B, Hunninghake R, Mikirova NA, Jackson JA, Gonzalez MJ, Miranda-Massari JR, Alexandrescu DT, Dasanu CA, Bogin V, Ancans J, Stevens RB, Markosian B, Koropatnick J, Chen CS, Riordan NH. Intravenous ascorbic acid to prevent and treat cancer-associated sepsis? J Transl Med. 2011;4(9):25.

22. Mikirova N, Casciari J, Rogers A, Taylor P. Effect of high-dose intravenous vitamin C on inflammation in cancer patients. J Transl Med. 2012;11(10):189.

23. Mikirova N, Hunninghake R. Effect of high dose vitamin C on Epstein-Barr viral infection. Med Sci Monit. 2014;3(20):725–32.

24. Pohanka M, Pejchal J, Snopkova S, Havlickova K, Karasova JZ, Bostik P, Pikula J. Ascorbic acid: an old player with a broad impact on body physiology including oxidative stress suppression and immunomodulation: a review. Mini Rev Med Chem. 2012 Jan;12(1):35-43. Review.

25. González MJ, Miranda-Massari JR, Mora EM, Guzmán A, Riordan NH, Riordan HD, Casciari JJ, Jackson JA, Román-Franco A. Orthomolecular oncology review: ascorbic acid and cancer 25 years later. Integr Cancer Ther. 2005 Mar;4(1):32-44. Review.

26. Hanahan D, Weinberg RA. Hallmarks of cancer: the next generation. Cell. 2011;144:646–74.

27. Moreno-Sánchez R, Rodríguez-Enríquez S, Marín-Hernández A, Saavedra E. Energy metabolism in tumor cells. FEBS J. 2007;274(6):1393–418.

28. Gonzalez MJ, Miranda Massari JR, Duconge J, Riordan NH, Ichim T, Quintero-Del-Rio AI, Ortiz N. The bio-energetic theory of carcinogenesis. Med Hypotheses. 2012 Oct;79(4):4339.

29. Xue J, Yang S, Seng S. Mechanisms of Cancer Induction by Tobacco-Specific NNK and NNN. Cancers (Basel). 2014;6(2):1138–56.

30. Varela-Rey M, Woodhoo A, Martinez-Chantar ML, Mato JM, Lu SC. Alcohol, DNA methylation, and cancer. Alcohol Res. 2013;35:25–35.
31. Alavanja MC, Ross MK, Bonner MR. Increased cancer burden among pesticide applicators and others due to pesticide exposure. CA Cancer J Clin. 2013;63(2):120–42.
32. Van Maele-Fabry G, Hoet P, Lison D. Parental occupational exposure to pesticides as risk factor for brain tumors in children and young adults: a systematic review and meta-analysis. Environ Int. 2013;56:19–31.
33. Arlt VM. 3-Nitrobenzanthrone, a potential human cancer hazard in diesel exhaust and urban air pollution: a review of the evidence. Mutagenesis. 2005;20:399–410.
34. Abnet CC. Carcinogenic food contaminants. Cancer Invest. 2007;25(3):189–96.
35. Sutandyo N. Nutritional carcinogenesis. Acta Med Indones. 2010;42(1):36–42.
36. Liu C, Russell RM. Nutrition and gastric cancer risk: an update. Nutr Rev. 2008;66(5):237–49.
37. Gach K, Wyrębska A, Fichna J, Janecka A. The role of morphine in regulation of cancer cell growth. Naunyn Schmiedebergs Arch Pharmacol. 2011;384:221–30.
38. Gong L, Dong C, Ouyang W, Qin Q. Regulatory T cells: a possible promising approach to cancer recurrence induced by morphine. Med Hypotheses. 2013;80:308–10.
39. Lennon FE, Moss J, Singleton PA. The µ-opioid receptor in cancer progression is there a direct effect? Anesthesiology. 2012;116:940–5.
40. King B, Jiang Y, Su X, Xu J, Xie L, Standard J, Wang W. Weight control, endocrine hormones and cancer prevention. Exp Biol Med. 2013;238:502–8.
41. Knower KC, To SQ, Leung YK, Ho SM, Clyne CD. Endocrine disruption of the epigenome: a breast cancer link. Endocr Relat Cancer. 2014;21(2):T33–55.
42. Sethi G, Shanmugam MK, Ramachandran L, Kumar AP, Tergaonkar V. Multifaceted link between cancer and inflammation. Biosci Rep. 2012;32:1–15.
43. Aggarwal BB, Gehlot P. Inflammation and cancer: how friendly is the relationship for cancer patients? Curr Opin Pharmacol. 2009;9:351–69.
44. Alibek K, Kakpenova A, Baiken Y. Role of infectious agents in the carcinogenesis of brain and head and neck cancers. Infect Agent Cancer. 2013;8:7.
45. Orlando A, Russo F. Intestinal microbiota, probiotics and human gastrointestinal cancers. J Gastrointest Cancer. 2013;44:121–31.
46. Reiche EM, Morimoto HK, Nunes SM. Stress and depression-induced immune dysfunction: implications for the development and progression of cancer. Int Rev Psychiatry. 2005;17:515–27.
47. Lillberg K, Verkasalo PK, Kaprio J, Teppo L, Helenius H, Koskenvuo M. Stressful life events and risk of breast cancer in 10,808 women: a cohort study. Am J Epidemiol. 2003;157:415–23.
48. Berrington de González A, Mahesh M, Kim KP, et al. Projected cancer risks from computed tomographic scans performed in the United States in 2007. Arch Intern Med. 2009 Dec 14;169(22):20717.
49. Anand P, Kunnumakara AB, Sundaram C, Harikumar KB, Tharakan ST, Lai OS, et al. Cancer is a preventable disease that requires major lifestyle changes. Pharm Res. 2008;25(9):2097–116.
50. Moen I, Stuhr LEB. Hyperbaric oxygen therapy and cancer—a review. Target Oncol. 2012;7(4): 233–242.
51. Bocci V, Larini A, Micheli V. Restoration of normoxia by ozone therapy may control neoplastic growth: a review and a working hypothesis. J Altern Complement Med. 2005;11(2):257–65.
52. Ciborowski M, Lipska A, Godzien J, Ferrarini A, Korsak J, Radziwon P, et al. Combination of LC-MS- and GC-MS-based metabolomics to study the effect of ozonated autohemotherapy on human blood. J Proteome Res. 2012;11(12):6231–41.
53. Wayner DDM, Burton GW, Ingold KU, Locke S. Quantitative measurement of the total, peroxyl radical-trapping antioxidant capability of human blood plasma by controlled peroxidation: The important contribution made by plasma proteins. FEBS. 1985;187:33–7.

54. Giunta R, Coppola A, Luongo C, Sammartino A, Guastafierro S, Grassia A, et al. Ozonized autohemotransfusion improves hemorheological parameters and oxygen delivery to tissues in patients with peripheral occlusive arterial disease. Ann Hematol. 2001;80(12):745–8.

55. Schulz S, Häussler U, Mandic R, Heverhagen JT, Neubauer A, Dünne AA, Werner JA, Weihe E, Bette M. Treatment with ozone/oxygen-pneumoperitoneum results in complete remission of rabbit squamous cell carcinomas. Int J Cancer. 2008;122(10):2360–7.

56. Gonzalez MJ. Lipid peroxidation and tumor growth: an inverse relationship. Med Hypotheses. 1992;38(2):106–10.

57. Stuhr LE, Raa A, Oyan AM, Kalland KH, Sakariassen PO, Petersen K, Bjerkvig R, Reed RK. Hyperoxia retards growth and induces apoptosis, changes in vascular density and gene expression in transplanted gliomas in nude rats. J Neurooncol. 2007;85:191–202.

58. Francescone R, Hou V, Grivennikov SI. Microbiome, inflammation, and cancer. Cancer J. 2014;20(3):181–9.

59. Robey IF, Baggett BK, Kirkpatrick ND, Roe DJ, Dosescu J, Sloane BF, Hashim AI, Morse DL, Raghunand N, Gatenby RA, Gillies RJ. Bicarbonate increases tumor pH and inhibits spontaneous metastases. Cancer Res. 2009;69(6):2260–8.

60. Robey IF, Martin NK. Bicarbonate and dichloroacetate: evaluating pH altering therapies in a mouse model for metastatic breast cancer. BMC Cancer. 2011;10(11):235.

61. Xie J, Wang BS, Yu DH, Lu Q, Ma J, Qi H, Fang C, Chen HZ. Dichloroacetate shifts the metabolism from glycolysis to glucose oxidation and exhibits synergistic growth inhibition with cisplatin in HeLa cells. Int J Oncol. 2011;38(2):409–17.

62. Agus DB, Vera JC, Golde DW. Stromal cell oxidation: a mechanism by which tumors obtain vitamin C. Cancer Res. 1999;59(18):4555–8.

63. Kc S, Cárcamo JM, Golde DW. Vitamin C enters mitochondria via facilitative glucose transporter 1 (Glut1) and confers mitochondrial protection against oxidative injury. FASEB J. 2005;19(12):1657–67.

64. McEligot AJ, Yang S, Meyskens FL Jr. Redox regulation by intrinsic species and extrinsic nutrients in normal and cancer cells. Annu Rev Nutr. 2005;25:26195. Review.

Index

© The Author(s) 2014
M.J. Gonzalez and J.R. Miranda-Massari, *New Insights on Vitamin C and Cancer*,
SpringerBriefs in Cancer Research, DOI 10.1007/978-1-4939-1890-4